PTCE® FLASHCARDS

Pharmacy Technician Certification Exam

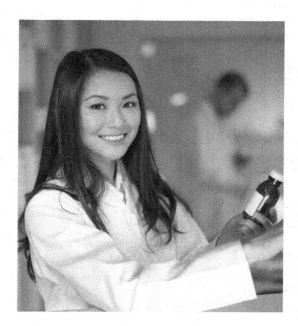

**Della Ata Khoury,
CPhT, MA, BS, BA**
Pharmacy Technician Instructor
LARE Training Center
Lawrence, Mass.

Research & Education Association
Visit our website at: www.rea.com

Research & Education Association
61 Ethel Road West
Piscataway, New Jersey 08854
E-mail: info@rea.com

Pharmacy Technician Certification Exam Flashcard Book with Online Practice

Printed in the United States of America

ISBN-13: 978-0-7386-1222-5
ISBN-10: 0-7386-1222-7

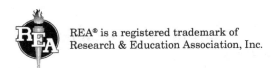

Table of Contents

A Note from the Author

As a pharmacy technician program instructor, I know that many pharmacy technician candidates like you are concerned about your readiness for the Pharmacy Technician Certification Exam (PTCE). You'll need to memorize a lot of terms, drug classifications, and other relevant information before test day. But don't worry—REA has designed this flashcard book, along with companion online assessment tools, to help you prepare completely for the exam.

As you begin your study, be sure to focus on the drug names. Because so many pharmacy technician preparation programs require their students to memorize the top 200 drug names, I've included them in this book. This flashcard book is a useful guide for learning about medications, their indications, interactions, side effects, and the appropriate auxiliary labels to use. Knowledge of these topics is emphasized in the new PTCE blueprint and it is also important on the job, as the scope of practice of pharmacy technicians continues to expand.

There is a high probability that out of the 90 multiple-choice PTCE questions, any medication-related question will be focused on the top 100 drug names. The first 100 flashcards in this book cover the top 100 drugs; don't underestimate the importance of learning those at a minimum.

As you prepare for the PTCE, it is critical to learn the major drug classifications and their associated side effects and interactions. To help you make the most of your study time, the drug-name flashcards show just the major side effects and interactions. The book also avoids bogging you down with a drug's off-label uses; for your purposes, it's important to familiarize yourself with only the primary uses of each drug.

The popular drug names covered in this book are written using the tall man lettering system, which uses uppercase letters to differentiate between sound-alike and look-alike drugs. In this case, I use tall man lettering to highlight the similarities in the prefixes or suffixes of drugs belonging to the same drug class. Noticing the similarities will help you master learning the drug names and their respective classifications.

When you take the actual PTCE, I recommend that you take your time and read all the answer choices carefully. Flag any questions you're unsure of. Review these questions if you have additional time. Do not leave any questions unanswered. If you absolutely cannot figure out a question, make an educated guess. Use any remaining time to review all your answers.

If you are comfortable with all the topics covered in this flashcard book, there is no reason why you can't pass the PTCE. Take your time preparing, review any areas where you feel you need extra practice, and relax before the exam.

Good luck on the PTCE!

Della Ata Khoury, CPhT, MA, BS, BA

Welcome to REA's PTCE Flashcard Book

Being a Pharmacy Technician is a rewarding career, and REA wants to help you succeed on the Pharmacy Technician Certification Exam (PTCE). Our flashcards are based on the content tested on the PTCE and will help you test your knowledge in all nine domains of the exam.

1. **This book includes 500 flashcards divided as follows:**

➡ 200 flashcards focused on the top 200 brand/generic drug names arranged in order by most popular drugs for 2015, including drug classes, indications, side effects, and special considerations

➡ 50 flashcards focused on pharmaceutical terms and abbreviations

➡ 250 flashcards focused on PTCE exam content and organized as follows:

- 165 flashcards on assisting the pharmacist in serving patients

- 55 flashcards on maintaining medication and inventory control systems

- 30 flashcards on participating in the administration and management of pharmacy practice

These flashcards include multiple-choice questions with detailed answer explanations and are similar to what you will encounter on the PTCE.

2. **The online REA Study Center includes:**

➡ 3 quizzes made up of questions from the book, with the added benefits of powerful scoring analysis and diagnostic tools that identify your strengths and weaknesses to help focus your study.

➡ e-flashcards

Use the REA Study Center to create your own unique flashcards, adding to the 150 e-flashcards included with this book. And, since you can access them online or on your smartphone, you can practice anytime you have a free moment.

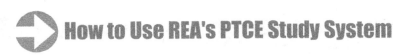

How to Use REA's PTCE Study System

There are many different ways to prepare for the PTCE. What's best for you depends on how much time you have to study and how comfortable you are with the subject matter. To score your highest, you need a study system that can be customized to fit you: your schedule, your learning style, and your current level of knowledge.

This flashcard book and the accompanying online tools will help you personalize your PTCE prep by testing your understanding, pinpointing your weaknesses, and delivering flashcard materials unique to you. REA's PTCE flashcards are an excellent way to refresh your knowledge and check your test-readiness before exam day.

Let's Get Started:

Review the Flashcards in the Book

Study the flashcards in the book. See how much you know about the content tested on the PTCE.

Test Yourself and Get Online Feedback

After you review with the book test yourself with our three quizzes available at the REA Study Center (*www.rea.com/studycenter*). These online quizzes are made up of questions from the book and have the added benefits of powerful scoring analysis and diagnostic tools that identify your strengths and weaknesses. Detailed score reports show you what you already know and pinpoint where you need to spend more time studying.

Improve Your Score with e-Flashcards

Armed with your score reports, you'll be able to see which areas you need to review. Use this information to create your own e-flashcards for the areas where you need additional practice. And, because you will create these flashcards through the REA Study Center, you'll be able to access them from any computer or smartphone.

Not sure what to put on your e-flashcards? Our PTCE e-flashcards come with 150 of the book's flashcards to get you started.

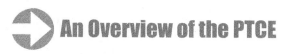# An Overview of the PTCE

The PTCE is made up of 90 multiple-choice questions, 10 of which are unscored and are included for evaluation purposes for possible inclusion on future exams. In effect, your score will be based on your answers to 80 questions. You need a minimum of 1400 points out of a total of 1600 to pass the test, or 87.5%, which is a minimum of 70 correct answers out of 80. You will have 120 minutes to complete the test.

The Pharmacy Technician Certification Board (PTCB) conducts a job analysis study approximately every five years. The results of the survey inform the construction of a new blueprint (content outline) for the PTCE. The PTCB introduced a new blueprint on November 1, 2013.

The blueprint organizes the test content into nine knowledge areas: Pharmacology for Technicians; Pharmacy Law and Regulations; Sterile and Nonsterile Compounding; Medication Safety; Pharmacy Quality Assurance; Medication Order Entry and Fill Process; Pharmacy Inventory Management; Pharmacy Billing and Reimbursement; and Pharmacy Information Systems Usage and Application. These knowledge areas are further divided into subcategories to convey more information about the content of the exam.

To learn more about the PTCE and register for the exam, contact:

Pharmacy Technician Certification Board
2215 Constitution Avenue NW
Washington, DC 20037
Phone: (800) 363-8012
www.ptcb.org
E-mail: contact@ptcb.org

About the Author

Della Ata Khoury holds a Master of Regional Economics and Social Development, a bachelor's degree in Political Science, and a bachelor's degree in Biological Sciences, all from the University of Massachusetts in Lowell. Della supplemented her education with practical experience, working as a hospital pharmacy technician for 12 years. In 2001, she obtained her national pharmacy certification through the Pharmacy Technician Certification Board (PTCB), becoming one of the earliest certified technicians in Massachusetts.

In 2010, Della moved on to instructing pharmacy technician programs at the LARE Institute in Andover Massachusetts (a branch of American Training) and Lincoln Technical Education in Somerville, Massachusetts. The classes included: Introduction to Fundamentals of Pharmacology, Pharmacy Law and Ethics, Medical and Pharmaceutical Terminology with Anatomy and Physiology, Asepsis and Infection Control, Pharmacology I, Drug Classifications, Pharmaceutical Compounding, Pharmacology II, Medication Calculations, Computers in Pharmacy, and Certification Exam Review.

To date, Della has taught for more than 5 years and more than 100 students. She has presented several continuing education topics specific to pharmacy technicians at national and state conferences. In 2015, she was one of just 14 outstanding writers chosen by the PTCB to participate in the Remote Item Writing Drive to develop new test content for the Pharmacy Technician Certification Exam.

Della has proudly achieved high success in student certification and job placement. She is a member of the Massachusetts Society of Health System Pharmacists (MSHP), the Pharmacy Technician Educators Council (PTEC), and the National Pharmacy Technician Association (NPTA).

About REA

Founded in 1959, Research & Education Association (REA) is dedicated to publishing the finest and most effective educational materials — including study guides and test preps — for students of all ages.

Today, REA's wide-ranging catalog is a leading resource for students, teachers, and other professionals. Visit *www.rea.com* to see a complete listing of all our titles.

Acknowledgments

In addition to our author, we would like to thank Pam Weston, Publisher, for setting the quality standards for production integrity and managing the publication to completion; Larry B. Kling, Vice President, Editorial, for his overall direction; Kelli Wilkins, Editor, for project management; John Paul Cording, Vice President, Technology, for coordinating the design and development of the online REA Study Center; Eve Grinnell, Graphic Designer, for cover design; and TCS for typesetting this edition.

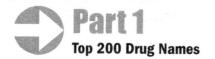
Brand names: Vicodin, Lortab, Lorcet Plus, Norco, Hycet, Anexsia, Xodol, Zamicet, Zydone

Generic name: Hydrocodone/acetaminophen

Drug class: Narcotic, analgesic

- Relieves pain.

(1)

Brand name: Nexium

Generic name: Esomeprazole

Drug class: Proton pump inhibitor (PPI)

- Prevents acid buildup.
- Notice the suffix *-prazole*, which distinguishes PPIs from other drug classes.

(2)

Indication: Moderate to moderately severe pain relief

Side effects: Drowsiness, sedation, dizziness

Special considerations:

- This is a Schedule II habit-forming drug. On October 6, 2014, the Drug Enforcement Agency (DEA) moved all hydrocodone-combination products to the Schedule II from the initial Schedule III category.

- The patient should not use in combination with acetaminophen or other products containing acetaminophen and to not exceed the maximum dose allowance of acetaminophen (doses that exceed 4 g of acetaminophen per day).

- The patient should not take with alcohol.

(1)

Indications: Gastroesophageal reflux disease (GERD), ulcers, heartburn

Side effects: Diarrhea, headache, hypertension, dizziness, nausea, abdominal pain, flatulence

Special considerations:

- The patient should not take if hypersensitive to other proton pump inhibitors.

- Medication should be taken 30–60 minutes prior to meal.

(2)

Brand names: OxyContin, Roxicodone, OxyIR, OxyFAST, Oxecta

Generic name: Oxycodone

Drug class: Opioid analgesic

- Relieves pain.

(3)

Brand name: Protonix

Generic name: Pantoprazole

Drug class: Proton pump inhibitor (PPI)

- Prevents acid buildup.
- Notice the suffix *-prazole*, which distinguishes PPIs from other drug classes.

(4)

Indication: Moderate to severe pain

Side effects: Nausea, vomiting, constipation, dizziness, sweating, flushing, weakness

Special considerations:

- This is a Schedule II habit-forming drug.
- The patient should not take with alcohol.

(3)

Indications: Gastroesophageal reflux disease (GERD), ulcers, heartburn

Side effects: Diarrhea, headache, hyperglycemia, nausea, abdominal pain, flatulence

Special considerations:

- The patient should not take if hypersensitive to other proton pump inhibitors.

(4)

Brand names: Prilosec, Zegerid

Generic name: Omeprazole

Drug class: Proton pump inhibitor (PPI)

- Prevents acid buildup.
- Notice the suffix *-prazole*, which distinguishes PPIs from other drug classes.

(5)

Brand name: Zocor

Generic name: Simvastatin

Drug class: Statin, HMG-CoA (3-hydroxy-3-methyl-glutaryl-CoA) reductase inhibitor

- Lowers low-density lipoprotein (LDL)/cholesterol.
- Notice the suffix *-statin*, which distinguishes lipid-lowering agents from other drug classes.

(6)

Indications: Gastroesophageal reflux disease (GERD), ulcers

Side effects: Diarrhea, headache, hyperglycemia, nausea, abdominal pain, flatulence

Special considerations:

- The patient should not take if hypersensitive to other proton pump inhibitors.

(5)

Indication: Hypercholesterolemia

Side effects: Constipation, flatulence, upper respiratory infection

Special considerations:

- The patient should avoid drinking more than one quart of grapefruit juice.
- This medication can lead to hepatic failure.

(6)

Brand name: Lipitor

Generic name: Atorvastatin

Drug class: Statin, HMG-CoA (3-hydroxy-3-methyl-glutaryl-CoA) reductase inhibitor, antilipemic

- Lowers low-density lipoprotein (LDL)/cholesterol (bad cholesterol).
- Notice the suffix -*statin*, which distinguishes lipid-lowering agents from other drug classes.

(7)

Brand name: Duragesic

Generic name: Fentanyl transdermal

Drug class: Opioid analgesic

- Relieves pain.

(8)

Indication: Hypercholesterolemia

Side effects: Myopathy, headache, chest pain, insomnia, dizziness, abdominal pain, constipation, diarrhea, dyspepsia, flatulence, arthralgia, sinusitis, flu-like symptoms

Special considerations:

- The patient should avoid drinking more than one quart of grapefruit juice per day and excessive alcohol consumption.
- This medication can be taken with food at any time of the day.
- Patients should be on a low-cholesterol diet prior to initiation of the medication and during therapy.
- Medication should be discontinued and the physician contacted immediately if the patient experiences muscle pain or brown urine.
- This medication is contraindicated in pregnancy.

(7)

Indication: Chronic pain

Side effects: Asthenia, confusion, constipation, dry mouth, nausea, vomiting

Special considerations:

- This is a Schedule II habit-forming drug.
- This medication has high potential for diversion.

(8)

Brand names: Zithromax, Zmax

Generic name: Azithromycin

Drug class: Macrolide antibiotic

- Stops bacterial growth by interfering with their ability to make protein.
- Notice the suffix *–romycin*, which distinguishes macrolide antibiotics from other drug classes.

(9)

Brand name: Valtrex

Generic name: Valacyclovir HCl

Drug class: Antiviral

- Treats viral infections.
- Notice the suffix *–vir*, which indicates that this drug is an antiviral.

(10)

Indications: Mild to moderate upper respiratory bacterial infections, acute sinusitis, acute otitis media, pharyngitis/ tonsillitis, pneumonia

Side effects: Diarrhea, nausea, abdominal pain

Special considerations:

- The patient should not take this medication with pimozide.
- The patient should complete the full course of therapy.

(9)

Indications: Herpes labialis (cold sores), herpes zoster, genital herpes

Side effects: Abdominal pain, headache, nausea

Special considerations:

- This medication may lead to acute renal failure in elderly patients or patients with renal impairment.

(10)

Brand name: Effexor ER

Generic name: Venlafaxine ER

Drug class: Antidepressant, serotonin–norepinephrine reuptake inhibitor (SNRI)

- Treats depression.

(11)

Brand name: Allegra

Generic name: Fexofenadine

Drug class: Antihistamine (2nd generation)

- Blocks the release of histamines.

(12)

Indications: Depression, generalized anxiety, social anxiety, panic disorder

Side effects: Headache, nausea, insomnia, asthenia, dizziness, dry mouth

Special considerations:

- This medication should not be taken concurrently with monoamine oxidase inhibitors (MAOIs).

- The patient should wait 14 days before initiating therapy after being on an MAOI or 7 days before taking an MAOI after stopping Effexor XR.

- Patients should be alerted that this medication should not be discontinued abruptly.

(11)

Indication: Seasonal allergies

Side effect: Headache

Special consideration:

- The patient should be aware that taking this medication with fruit juice may decrease its efficacy.

(12)

Brand names: Neurontin, Gralise, Horizant

Generic name: Gabapentin

Drug class: Anticonvulsant

- Treats seizures.

(13)

Brand names: Percocet, Tylox, Primlev, Roxicet

Generic name: Oxycodone/acetaminophen

Drug class: Narcotic, analgesic, antipyretic

- Relieves pain and reduces fever.

(14)

Indications: Epilepsy, neuropathic pain

Side effects: Ataxia, dizziness, fatigue, somnolence

Special considerations:

- Patients should be alerted that this medication should not be discontinued abruptly.

- The patient should not take this medication with alcohol.

(13)

Indication: Moderate to moderately severe pain relief

Side effects: Lightheadedness, dizziness, drowsiness or sedation, nausea, vomiting

Special considerations:

- This medication is a Schedule II habit-forming drug.

- The patient should not use this medication in combination with acetaminophen or other products containing acetaminophen in order to not exceed the maximum dose allowance of acetaminophen (doses that exceed 4 g of acetaminophen per day).

- The patient should not take this medication with alcohol.

(14)

Brand names: Zestril, Prinivil

Generic name: Lisinopril

Drug class: Angiotensin converting enzyme (ACE) inhibitor

- Decreases blood pressure and dilates blood vessels.

(15)

Brand name: Plavix

Generic name: Clopidogrel

Drug class: Antiplatelet agent, platelet inhibitor

- Stops platelets from aggregating.

(16)

Indications: Hypertension, heart failure

Side effects: Dizziness, cough, headache

Special consideration:

- Alert pharmacist if a patient on an ACE inhibitor attempts to buy cough medication or complains of a cough. The cessation of the treatment is the only effective treatment for the ACE inhibitor-related cough.

(15)

Indication: Reduces possibility of atherothrombotic events in patients who recently experienced stroke or peripheral arterial disease

Side effects: Bleeding, abdominal pain, vomiting, dyspepsia, gastritis, constipation, chest pain, edema, dizziness, rash

Special considerations:

- This medication is usually taken around the same time once a day with or without food.

- Avoid anticoagulants, antiplatelet agents, NSAIDs, salicylates, thrombolytics, and other blood-thinning medication.

(16)

Brand name: Prevacid

Generic name: Lansoprazole

Drug class: Proton pump inhibitor (PPI)

- Prevents acid buildup.
- Notice the suffix *-prazole*, which distinguishes PPIs from other drug classes.

(17)

Brand names: Levoxyl, Synthroid, L Thyroxine, Levo T, Levothroid, Levoxine, Tirosint, Unithroid

Generic name: Levothyroxine

Drug class: Thyroid hormone, antihypothyroid

- Replaces thyroid hormone.

(18)

Indications: Gastroesophageal reflux disease (GERD), ulcers, heartburn

Side effects: Diarrhea, nausea, headache, fatigue, abdominal pain

Special consideration:

- The patient should not take this medication if hypersensitive to other proton pump inhibitors.

(17)

Indications: Hypothyroidism, goiter

Side effects: Arrhythmias, cramps, diarrhea, nervousness, tachycardia, tremor

Special considerations:

- This medication should not be used for treatment of obesity or for weight loss.
- The patient should not take this medication if allergic to aspirin.

(18)

Brand name: Singulair

Generic name: Montelukast

Drug class: Anti-asthmatic, leukotriene receptor inhibitor

- Blocks bronchorestriction effects of leukotrienes, thereby producing bronchodilation.

(19)

Brand name: Norvasc

Generic name: Amlodipine besylate

Drug class: Calcium channel blocker

- Decreases blood pressure.

(20)

Indications: Prophylactic and chronic treatment of asthma

Side effects: Abdominal pain, dizziness, myalgia, headache, fatigue, fever, dyspepsia, gastroenteritis, cough, nasal congestion, weakness

Special considerations:

- Patient should take medication once a day in the evening.
- Patient should avoid taking aspirin and NSAIDs while on this medication.

(19)

Indications: Hypertension, angina

Side effects: Edema, headache, fatigue, palpitation, dizziness, flushing, nausea

Special consideration:

- The prescriber needs to adjust the dose for patients with severe hepatic impairment because this medication is extensively metabolized by the liver.

(20)

Brand names: Flonase, Veramyst

Generic name: Fluticasone intranasal

Drug class: Corticosteroid, intranasal

- Reduces inflammation and mucus production.

(21)

Brand names: Xanax, Niravam

Generic name: Alprazolam

Drug class: Benzodiazepine

- Produces sedation, induces sleep (hypnotic), reduces anxiety (anxiolytic), reduces convulsions (anticonvulsant), and relaxes muscles.

- Notice the suffix *-olam*, which distinguishes benzodiazepines from other drug classes.

(22)

Indications: Allergic and nonallergic nasal symptoms

Side effects: Headache, upper respiratory infection, pharyngitis, nasal congestion, nasal discharge, allergic rhinitis, dysphonia

Special considerations:

- Patients with recent nasal injury or surgery should avoid this medication.

(21)

Indications: Anxiety, panic disorders

Side effects: Drowsiness, depression, headache, constipation, diarrhea, dry mouth

Special considerations:

- This is a Schedule IV habit-forming drug.
- This medication should not be taken with alcohol.
- Patients should be alerted to not discontinue this medication abruptly.

(22)

Brand name: Flomax

Generic name: Tamsulosin HCl

Drug class: Alpha blocker or alpha antagonist

- Blocks alpha receptors, resulting in vasoconstriction and decreased gastrointestinal motility.

(23)

Brand name: Crestor

Generic name: Rosuvastatin

Drug class: Statin, HMG-CoA (3-hydroxy-3-methyl-glutaryl-CoA) reductase inhibitor

- Lowers low-density lipoprotein (LDL)/cholesterol
- Notice the suffix -*statin*, which distinguishes lipid-lowering agents from other drug classes.

(24)

Indication: Benign prostatic hypertrophy (BPH)

Side effects: Hypotension, dizziness, gastrointestinal upset, nasal congestion, drowsiness

Special considerations:

- The first dose of this medication may cause loss of consciousness. The patient should be alerted to avoid standing up quickly upon initiation of this medication.

- This medication should not be taken with alcohol.

(23)

Indication: Hypercholesterolemia

Side effects: Constipation, flatulence, upper respiratory infection

Special considerations:

- The patient should avoid excessive drinking of alcohol and grapefruit juice.

- This medication can be taken any time of the day.

- The medication should be discontinued and the physician contacted immediately if the patient experiences muscle pain or brown urine.

- This medication is contraindicated in pregnancy.

(24)

Brand names: Glucophage, Fortamet, Glumetza, Riomet

Generic name: Metformin

Drug class: Antihyperglycemic

- Controls blood sugar by decreasing hepatic glucose production, decreasing glucose absorption by the gastrointestinal system, and improves target cell response to insulin.

(25)

Brand name: Zoloft

Generic name: Sertraline

Drug class: Selective serotonin reuptake inhibitor (SSRI), antidepressant

- Treats depression.

(26)

Indication: Type 2 diabetes mellitus (non-insulin-dependent diabetes)

Side effects: Asthenia, diarrhea, flatulence, gastrointestinal complaints, nausea, vomiting

Special consideration:

- Patients with hepatic disease and patients aged 80 years or older with renal impairment should avoid this medication.

(25)

Indications: Depression, panic disorder, obsessive-compulsive disorder (OCD)

Side effects: Diarrhea, nausea, headache, insomnia, dizziness, dry mouth, fatigue, somnolence

Special considerations:

- This medication is not approved for use in pediatric patients.

- Patients must allow a 14-day withdrawal period before or after taking a monoamine oxidase inhibitor (MAOI).

(26)

Brand name: Lopressor

Generic name: Metoprolol tartrate

Drug class: Beta blocker, beta$_1$ selective blocker

- Blocks action of epinephrine and norepinephrine on beta receptors located mainly in the heart and kidneys.

- Notice the suffix *-olol*, which distinguishes beta blockers from other drug classes.

(27)

Brand name: Omnicef

Generic name: Cefdinir

Drug class: Cephalosporin antibiotic

- Kills bacteria by interfering with their cell wall formation.

- Notice the prefix *cef-*, which distinguishes cephalosporins from other drug classes.

(28)

Indications: Acute myocardial infarction, congestive heart failure (CHF), hypertension, angina

Side effects: Dizziness, headache, tiredness, depression, diarrhea, pruritus, bradycardia, dyspnea, cold extremities, constipation, dyspepsia, heart failure, hypotension, nausea, wheezing

Special considerations:

- Patients should not take this medication concurrently with other beta blockers.

- Patients should be aware that this medication should not be discontinued abruptly without the recommendation of a physician.

- This medication is not interchangeable with metoprolol succinate (Toprol XL).

(27)

Indications: Community-acquired pneumonia, respiratory tract infections, acute maxillary sinusitis, skin infections

Side effects: Diarrhea, nausea, rash, headache

Special consideration:

- The prescriber should reduce the dose by half in patients with renal impairment.

(28)

Brand name: Cozaar

Generic name: Losartan potassium

Drug class: Angiotensin receptor blocker (ARB)

- Notice the suffix -*sartan*, which distinguishes ARBs from other drug classes.

(29)

Brand name: Risperdal

Generic name: Risperidone

Drug class: Antipsychotic (2nd generation)

- Treats psychosis by tranquilizing the patient.

(30)

Indication: Hypertension

Side effects: Fatigue, hypoglycemia, chest pain, cough, diarrhea, upper respiratory infection, hypotension, dizziness, nausea

Special considerations:

- Patients should not use this medication if pregnant.

- The patients should be alerted not to take this medication concurrently with ACE inhibitors and beta-adrenergic blocking agents.

(29)

Indications: Schizophrenia, bipolar mania

Side effects: Somnolence, insomnia, agitation, anxiety, headache, rhinitis, constipation, dyspepsia, nausea, vomiting

Special consideration:

- This medication is not approved for treatment of patients with dementia-related psychosis.

(30)

Brand name: Pravachol

Generic name: Pravastatin

Drug class: Statin, HMG-CoA (3-hydroxy-3-methyl-glutaryl-CoA) reductase inhibitor

- Reduces low-density lipoprotein (LDL)/cholesterol.
- Notice the suffix *-statin*, which distinguishes lipid-lowering agents from other drug classes.

(31)

Brand names: Amoxil, Moxatag, Trimox

Generic name: Amoxicillin

Drug class: Penicillin antibiotic

- Kills bacteria by interfering with their cell wall formation.

(32)

Indication: Hypercholesterolemia or hyperlipidemia

Side effects: Nausea, vomiting, diarrhea, headache, chest pain, fatigue, rash, cough, heartburn, myalgia

Special considerations:

- The patient should be aware that there is a risk of rhabdomyolysis with taking this medication. If myopathy develops, the patient should discontinue the medication.

- Patients with active liver disease should avoid this medication.

(31)

Indications: Bacterial infections, strep throat, gonorrhea, anthrax prophylaxis, endocarditis prophylaxis

Side effects: Anaphylaxis, anemia, candidiasis, diarrhea, headache, nausea, rash, vomiting

Special consideration:

- The patient should not take this medication if allergic to penicillins, cephalosporins, or carbapenems.

(32)

Brand names: Depakote, Depakene, Depacon, Deproic, Stavzor

Generic name: Valproic acid

Drug class: Anticonvulsant

- Reduces seizures.

(33)

Brand name: Lexapro

Generic name: Escitalopram

Drug class: Selective serotonin reuptake inhibitor (SSRI), antidepressant

- Treats depression.

(34)

Indications: Partial seizures, migraine prophylaxis, bipolar mania

Side effects: Nausea, increased bleeding time, thrombocytopenia, tremor, asthenia, infection, somnolence, amblyopia, diarrhea, diplopia, dizziness, dyspepsia, nystagmus, tinnitus, vomiting

Special considerations:

- Patients should be aware that this medication has black box warnings because it may lead to hepatotoxicity, teratogenicity, and pancreatitis.

- Patients with liver disease should avoid this medication.

(33)

Indications: Depression, generalized anxiety disorder

Side effects: Headache, somnolence, insomnia, nausea, chest pain, hypertension, drowsiness, dizziness, fatigue, decreased libido, diarrhea, decreased appetite, constipation, rhinitis, flu-like syndrome

Special considerations:

- This medication should be taken once daily with or without food.

- Patients should not discontinue this medication abruptly.

- Patients must allow a 14-day withdrawal period before or after taking a monoamine oxidase inhibitor (MAOI).

(34)

Brand names: Prozac, Sarafem, Selfemra

Generic name: Fluoxetine

Drug class: Selective serotonin reuptake inhibitor (SSRI), antidepressant

- Treats depression.

(35)

Brand names: Ambien, Edluar, Intermezzo, Zolpimist

Generic name: Zolpidem tartrate

Drug class: Sedative, hypnotic

- Produces sedation and induces sleep.

(36)

Indications: Major depressive disorder, obsessive-compulsive disorder, bulimia nervosa, panic disorder, premenstrual dysphoric disorder

Side effects: Headache, nausea, insomnia, anorexia, anxiety, asthenia, diarrhea, nervousness, somnolence, dizziness, dry mouth, dyspepsia, sweating, tremor, decreased libido

Special considerations:

- Patients should be aware that this medication has a black box warning because of the increased risk of suicidal thoughts and behavior in anyone under the age of 24.

- The drug should not be used in pediatric patients.

- This medication should not be taken at the same time as MAOIs.

- Patients should not abruptly stop this medication; the dose is gradually discontinued.

(35)

Indication: Insomnia

Side effects: Dizziness, headache, somnolence, allergy, asthenia, constipation, depression, diarrhea, drowsiness, dry mouth, hallucinations, lightheadedness, memory disorder, myalgia

Special considerations:

- This medication is a Schedule IV controlled substance.

- Patients on this medication should avoid use of alcohol and other CNS depressants.

(36)

Brand name: ProAir HFA, Ventolin HFA, Proventil HFA

Generic name: Albuterol

Drug class: Bronchodilator, antiasthmatic, short-acting $beta_2$ agonist

- Increases airflow to the lungs by dilating the bronchi and bronchioles.
- MDI and nebulizer solution are available.

(37)

Brand name: Diovan

Generic name: Valsartan

Drug class: Angiotensin receptor blocker (ARB)

- Notice the suffix *-sartan*, which distinguishes ARBs from other drug classes.

(38)

Indications: Treatment or prevention of bronchospasms, prophylaxis for exercise-induced asthma

Side effects: Bronchospasm, tremor, nervousness, low potassium, high blood pressure, mild nausea and vomiting, headache, dizziness, cough, dry mouth and throat, insomnia, muscle pain, diarrhea

Special considerations:

- There is a risk of hypokalemia with use of this medication.
- This medication is contraindicated in patients with tachycardia associated with a heart condition.
- Hydrofluoroalkane (HFA) is the propellant in the inhaler.

(37)

Indications: Hypertension, treatment of heart failure

Side effects: Fatigue, hypoglycemia, chest pain, cough, diarrhea, upper respiratory infection, hypotension, dizziness, nausea

Special considerations:

- Patients should not use this medication if pregnant.
- Efficacy may be decreased with use of amphetamines and NSAIDs.

(38)

Brand names: Mevacor, Altoprev

Generic name: Lovastatin

Drug class: Statin, HMG-CoA (3-hydroxy-3-methyl-glutaryl-CoA) reductase inhibitor

- Reduces low-density lipoprotein (LDL)/cholesterol.

- Notice the suffix *-statin*, which distinguishes lipid-lowering agents from other drug classes.

(39)

Brand names: Cardizem CD, Cardizem LA, Cartia XT, Dilacor, Dilatrate, Diltiazem, Dilt-CD, Diltia XT, Diltiaz, Dilzem, Taztia XT, Tiazac

Generic name: Diltiazem CD

Drug class: Calcium channel blocker

- Decreases blood pressure.

(40)

Indication: Hypercholesterolemia

Side effects: Flatulence, abdominal pain, constipation, diarrhea, myalgia, nausea, dyspepsia, weakness, blurred vision, rash, muscle cramps, dizziness

Special considerations:

- This medication is contraindicated in pregnancy, hypersensitivity to statins, heavy alcohol use, renal failure, and liver disease.

- Patients should be aware that there is a risk of myopathy with taking this medication.

- Extended-release lovastatin should not be used concomitantly with cyclosporine.

(39)

Indications: Hypertension, angina, paroxysmal supraventricular tachycardia (PSVT), atrial fibrillation, atrial flutter

Side effects: Edema, headache, dizziness, atrioventricular (AV) block, peripheral edema, bradyarrhythmia, headache, hypotension, nausea, congestive heart failure, syncope, gingival hyperplasia

Special considerations:

- This medication should not be used by patients with AV block, hypotension, persistent/progressive dermatologic reactions, and hepatic/renal impairment.

- This medication should not be used concurrently with clonidine.

(40)

Brand names: Ultram, Rybix ODT, Ryzolt

Generic name: Tramadol

Drug class: Opioid analgesic

- Relieves pain by acting on the central nervous system.

(41)

Indication: Moderate to severe pain

Side effects: Dizziness, vertigo, constipation, nausea, headache, somnolence, vomiting, pruritus, agitation, anxiety, emotional lability, euphoria, hallucinations, nervousness, spasticity, asthenia, dyspepsia, sweating, diarrhea, dry mouth, hypertonia, malaise, menopausal symptoms, rash, urinary retention, urinary frequency, vasodilation, visual disturbance

Special considerations:

- This medication should not be used by patients with hypersensitivity to tramadol or opioids, acute intoxication with alcohol, suicidal patients, and opioid dependency.

- Patients should not use this medication concurrently with hypnotics, centrally acting analgesics, opioids, or psychotropic drugs.

- This medication has a risk of seizures that increases with doses that are above the recommended range.

- This medication should not be coadministered with serotonergic drugs.

- As of August 18, 2014, tramadol has been placed in Schedule IV nationally.

(41)

Brand name: Cymbalta

Generic name: Duloxetine

Drug class: Antidepressant, serotonin-norepinephrine reuptake inhibitor (SNRI)

- Treats depression.

(42)

Brand name: Seroquel

Generic name: Quetiapine

Drug class: Antipsychotic (2nd generation)

(43)

Indications: Depression, generalized anxiety, social anxiety, panic disorder

Side effects: Headache, somnolence, nausea, insomnia, dizziness, diarrhea, constipation, fatigue, anxiety, decreased libido, decreased appetite, muscle cramping

Special considerations:

- This medication should not be taken concurrently with monoamine oxidase inhibitors (MAOIs).

- The patient should wait 14 days before initiating therapy after being on an MAOI or 7 days before taking an MAOI after stopping medication.

- The patient should not discontinue this medication abruptly.

(42)

Indications: Schizophrenia, bipolar mania, depressive episodes

Side effects: Hypotension, somnolence, sedation, headache, agitation, dizziness, extrapyramidal symptoms, increase in cholesterol, weight gain, fatigue, pain, lethargy, weakness, anxiety, pharyngitis, nasal congestion, rhinitis

Special considerations:

- Patients should not take this medication in higher doses or for longer than recommended by the physician.

- This medication is not approved for treatment of patients with dementia-related psychosis.

- This medication may be sedating and may induce orthostatic hypotension.

- New or worsening symptoms should be reported to the physician.

(43)

Brand name: Celexa

Generic name: Citalopram HBR

Drug class: Selective serotonin reuptake inhibitor (SSRI), antidepressant

- Treats depression.

(44)

Brand name: Ativan

Generic name: Lorazepam

Drug class: Benzodiazepine, anticonvulsant, antianxiety agent, anxiolytic

- Produces sedation, induces sleep (hypnotic), reduces anxiety (anxiolytic), reduces seizures (anticonvulsant), and relaxes muscles.

- Notice the suffix -*am*, which distinguishes benzodiazepines from other drug classes.

(45)

Indication: Depression

Side effects: Dry mouth, nausea, somnolence, insomnia, increased sweating, tremor, diarrhea, rhinitis, upper respiratory infection, dyspepsia, fatigue, vomiting, anxiety, anorexia, abdominal pain, agitation, impotence, sinusitis, dysmenorrheal, decreased libido, arthralgia, myalgia

Special considerations:

- Patients should be aware that this medication has a black box warning due to its increased risk of suicidal thoughts and behavior in anyone under the age of 24.

- The drug should not be used in pediatric patients.

- This medication should not be used concomitantly with pimozide, NSAIDs, anticoagulants, MAO inhibitors, and other serotonergic drugs.

(44)

Indications: Anxiety, insomnia (short-term), preoperative sedation

Side effects: Sedation, dizziness, weakness, unsteadiness

Special considerations:

- This is a Schedule IV habit-forming drug.

- This medication should not be taken with alcohol.

- Patients on this medication for a prolonged time should be withdrawn gradually.

(45)

Brand names: Coumadin, Jantoven

Generic name: Warfarin

Drug class: Anticoagulant

- Prevents blood clot formation.

(46)

Brand names: Phenergan, Phenadoz, Promethegan

Generic name: Promethazine

Drug class: Phenothiazine, antihistamine, antiemetic, sedative

- Blocks the effects of histamines.

(47)

Indications: Deep venous thrombosis, atrial fibrillation, cardiac valve replacement, postmyocardial infarction

Side effects: Bleeding and hemorrhage

Special considerations:

- This drug interacts with a lot of drug classes including: anticoagulants, antiplatelet agents, nonsteroidal anti-inflammatory drugs (NSAIDs), antifungals, and selective serotonin reuptake inhibitors (SSRIs).

- Patients should be instructed to immediately report signs or symptoms of bleeding to their physician.

- All treated patients should have regular monitoring of the international normalized ratio (INR), which determines the clotting ability of the blood.

(46)

Indications: Allergy symptoms, motion sickness, postoperation nausea and vomiting

Side effects: Bradycardia, hypertension, postural hypotension, tachycardia, confusion, delirium, disorientation, dizziness

Special considerations:

- This medication may be sedating.

- Patients should be cautioned that this medication may impair their physical and mental abilities.

(47)

Brand name: Lotensin

Generic name: Benazepril

Drug class: Angiotensin-converting enzyme (ACE) inhibitor

- Decreases blood pressure and dilates blood vessels.

(48)

Brand name: Klonopin

Generic name: Clonazepam

Drug class: Benzodiazepine, anticonvulsant, antianxiety, anxiolytic

- Produces sedation, induces sleep (hypnotic), reduces anxiety (anxiolytic), reduces seizures (anticonvulsant), and relaxes muscles.

- Notice the suffix *-pam*, which distinguishes benzodiazepines from other drug classes.

(49)

Indications: Hypertension, heart failure

Side effects: Dizziness, cough, headache, fatigue, somnolence, nausea, hyperkalemia

Special considerations:

- Alert pharmacist if a patient on an ACE inhibitor attempts to buy cough medication or complains of a cough. The cessation of the treatment is the only effective treatment for the ACE inhibitor-related cough.

- This medication is contraindicated in pregnancy.

(48)

Indications: Seizures and panic disorders

Side effects: Somnolence, abnormal coordination, ataxia, depression, dizziness, fatigue, memory impairment, upper respiratory infection, confusion, dysarthria, rhinitis, coughing, urinary frequency, impotence, decreased libido

Special considerations:

- This is a Schedule IV habit-forming drug.

- This medication should not be taken with alcohol.

- This medication is contraindicated in patients with significant hepatic impairment, documented hypersensitivity, acute alcohol intoxication, myasthenia gravis, and severe respiratory depression.

- This medication should not be stopped abruptly when used for panic disorder.

(49)

Brand name: Fosamax

Generic name: Alendronate

Drug class: Calcium metabolism modifiers

- Prevents osteoporosis in postmenopausal women.

(50)

Brand names: Microzide, Oretic, HydroDiuril, Hydro, Esidrix

Generic name: Hydrochlorothiazide (HCTZ)

Drug class: Thiazide diuretic

- Increases fluid excretion.

(51)

Indication: Osteoporosis

Side effects: Hypercalcemia, abdominal pain, abdominal distention, acid regurgitation, bone/muscle/joint pain, constipation, diarrhea, dyspepsia, esophagitis, flatulence, headache, hypophosphatemia, musculoskeletal pain, nausea

Special considerations:

- This medication should be taken with plenty of water only.

- Patients on this medication should ensure adequate intake of calcium and vitamin D.

- Patients should be instructed to contact their physician if they develop symptoms of esophagitis.

(50)

Indications: Excess fluid buildup in the body (edema), hypertension

Side effects: Anorexia, epigastric distress, hypokalemia, hypotension, phototoxicity

Special considerations:

- This medication may lead to sensitivity reactions with or without history of allergy or asthma.

- Patients with history of sulfonamide or penicillin allergy should avoid this medication.

(51)

Brand names: Imitrex, Sumavel DosePro, Alsuma

Generic name: Sumatriptan oral

Drug class: Serotonin 5-HT-receptor agonist

- Activates serotonin receptors, resulting in a decrease of migraine headaches.

(52)

Brand name: Mirapex

Generic name: Pramipexole dihydrochloride

Drug class: Antiparkinson, dopamine agonist

- Acts on dopamine receptors and is used to treat the symptoms of Parkinson's disease.

(53)

Indication: Migraine headache

Side effects: Paresthesia, chest, jaw or neck tightness, fatigue, warm/cold sensation

Special considerations:

- This medication should not be used within 2 weeks of MAO inhibitors or within 24 hours of ergot-type medications.

- This medication may cause rebound migraine with overuse; use should be limited to 2 days per week.

- Patients using this medication should not take it concurrently with SSRIs.

(52)

Indications: Parkinson's disease, restless legs syndrome

Side effects: Somnolence, dyskinesia, hallucinations, insomnia, dizziness, nausea, constipation

Special considerations:

- Patients who develop sudden daytime "sleep attacks" should discontinue this medication.

- This medication should be gradually discontinued.

- Extended-release tablets should not be chewed, crushed, or divided.

(53)

Brand name: Coreg

Generic name: Carvedilol

Drug class: Beta blocker

- Blocks action of epinephrine and norepinephrine on both beta receptors and alpha$_1$ receptors.

- Notice the suffix *-lol*, which distinguishes beta blockers from other drug classes.

(54)

Brand name: Spiriva

Generic name: Tiotropium

Drug class: Anticholinergic

(55)

Indications: Congestive heart failure (CHF), hypertension (HTN), left ventricular dysfunction following myocardial infarction

Side effects: Dizziness, fatigue, hypotension, hyperglycemia, weight gain, diarrhea, bradycardia, cough, headache, atrioventricular block, edema, angina, vomiting, dyspnea, syncope, nausea, rhinitis

Special considerations:

- This medication should not be used by patients with bronchial asthma, bronchospasm, and sinus bradycardia.

- This medication should not be discontinued abruptly.

- Patients on Coreg CR should separate intake of any form of alcohol by at least 2 hours.

(54)

Indication: Treatment of bronchospasm associated with chronic obstructive pulmonary disease (COPD)

Side effects: Dry mouth, upper respiratory tract infection, sinusitis, pharyngeal irritation, edema, angina, rash, dyspepsia, abdominal pain, constipation, vomiting, urinary tract infection, myalgia, pharyngitis, rhinitis

Special considerations:

- Patients should be aware that this medication contains lactose.

(55)

Brand name: Abilify

Generic name: Aripiprazole

Drug class: Atypical antipsychotic

(56)

Brand name: Tenormin

Generic name: Atenolol

Drug class: Beta blocker, beta$_1$ selective blocker

- Blocks action of epinephrine and norepinephrine on beta receptors located mainly in the heart and kidneys.

- Notice the suffix *-olol*, which distinguishes beta blockers from other drug classes.

(57)

Indications: Schizophrenia, bipolar disorder, depression

Side effects: Headache, agitation, anxiety, insomnia, extrapyramidal symptoms, somnolence, dizziness, edema, dyspepsia, hypertension, tremor, weakness, myalgia, blurred vision, rhinitis, pharyngitis, cough

Special considerations:

- Patients should avoid alcohol.

- Patients should not discontinue this medication abruptly.

- Although this medication ends in the suffix –*prazole*, it is not a proton pump inhibitor.

(56)

Indications: Hypertension, acute myocardial infarction, angina

Side effects: Tiredness, bradycardia, hypotension, dizziness, cold extremities, fatigue, dyspnea, nausea, postural hypotension, bradycardia, wheeziness, diarrhea, lethargy, lightheadedness, drowsiness, vertigo

Special considerations:

- The patient should not take concurrently with other beta blockers.

- This medication should not be abruptly discontinued.

(57)

Brand name: Lovenox

Generic name: Enoxaparin sodium

Drug class: Anticoagulant

- Reduces the risk of developing blood clots.

(58)

Brand names: Medrol, Depo-Medrol

Generic name: Methylprednisolone

Drug class: Corticosteroid

- Exhibits anti-inflammatory effects.

(59)

Indications: Deep vein thrombosis, unstable angina, treatment of acute ST-segment elevation myocardial infarction (STEMI)

Side effects: Hemorrhage, elevation of serum aminotransferases, fever, local site reactions, thrombocytopenia, nausea, anemia, ecchymosis

Special considerations:

- Patients should be aware that this medication should not be administered intramuscularly (IM).

- This medication should not be used concomitantly with NSAIDs, platelet inhibitors, and other anticoagulants.

(58)

Indications: Allergies, asthma, arthritis

Side effects: Adrenal suppression, edema, hypertension, arrhythmia, insomnia, nervousness, psychosis, vertigo, headache, hallucinations, nausea, vomiting, increased appetite, hirsutism, acne, osteoporosis, myopathy, delayed wound healing

Special considerations:

- Patients should be aware that this medication is not indicated for long-term treatment.

- This medication should be taken with food or after a meal.

(59)

Brand names: Paxil, Pexeva

Generic name: Paroxetine

Drug class: Selective serotonin reuptake inhibitor (SSRI), antidepressant

- Treats depression.

(60)

Brand names: Keflex, Panixine Disperdose

Generic name: Cephalexin

Drug class: 1st-generation cephalosporin antibiotic

- Kills bacteria by interfering with their cell wall formation.
- The prefixes *cef-* or *ceph-* distinguish cephalosporins from other drug classes.

(61)

Indications: Depression, obsessive-compulsive disorder, generalized anxiety disorder, panic disorders

Side effects: Nausea, somnolence, insomnia, dry mouth, headache, asthenia, constipation, diarrhea, dizziness, sweating, tremor, anxiety, blurred vision, decrease in appetite, impotence, nervousness

Special considerations:

- Patients should be aware that this medication has a black box warning due to its increased risk of suicidal thoughts and behavior in anyone under the age of 24.

- The drug should not be used in pediatric patients.

- This medication should not be taken at the same time as MAOIs and other serotonergic drugs.

- Patients should not abruptly stop this medication; the dose is gradually discontinued.

(60)

Indication: Bacterial infections

Side effects: Abdominal pain, diarrhea, hypersensitivity

Special consideration:

- Patients should be aware that they must finish the full course of therapy unless otherwise indicated by their physician.

(61)

Brand names: Proscar, Propecia

Generic name: Finasteride

Drug class: Antiandrogen, 5-alpha-reductase inhibitor

- Blocks the action of androgen hormones.

(62)

Brand names: Concerta, Daytrana, Metadate CD, Metadate ER, Methylin, Methylin ER, Ritalin, Ritalin LA, Ritalin-SR

Generic name: Methylphenidate

Drug class: Central nervous system stimulant

- Excites the nervous system.

(63)

Indications: Benign prostatic hyperplasia (BPH)—enlarged prostate, androgenic alopecia

Side effects: Rash, breast tenderness/enlargement, decreased libido, impotence

Special considerations:

- Technicians should be aware that pregnant and potentially pregnant women should not handle crushed or broken tablets. This medication can lead to birth defects in sex organs of unborn male fetus.

(62)

Indications: Narcolepsy, attention deficit hyperactivity disorder (ADHD)

Side effects: Dizziness, hypertension, insomnia, decreased appetite, tic, emotional instability, vomiting, anorexia, nasal congestion, nasopharyngitis

Special considerations:

- This is a Schedule II habit-forming drug.

- The patient should not take concurrently with monoamine oxidase inhibitors (MAOIs).

- Patients with hypertension and advanced arteriosclerosis should avoid this medication.

(63)

Brand name: Lanoxin

Generic name: Digoxin

Drug class: Cardiac glycoside, inotrope, antiarrhythmic

- Improves the efficiency of the heart's action by decreasing the heart rate and increasing cardiac output.

(64)

Brand names: Namenda, Ebixa

Generic name: Memantine

Drug class: Anti-Alzheimer's, N-methyl-D-aspartate antagonist

- Treats moderate to severe Alzheimer's disease.

(65)

Indications: Congestive heart failure, atrial fibrillation, atrial flutter, tachycardia, cardiogenic shock (when the blood pumped by the heart does not meet the body's need)

Side effects: Heart block, headache, dizziness, mental disturbances, confusion, nausea, vomiting, diarrhea, abdominal pain, weakness

Special considerations:

- This medication should not be taken concurrently with a high-fiber meal. The patient should allow 1 hour before or 2 hours after such a meal.

- This medication should not be stopped unless advised by a physician.

(64)

Indications: Dementia associated with Alzheimer's disease

Side effects: Hypertension, dizziness, drowsiness, confusion, headache, hallucinations, pain, somnolence, fatigue, constipation, vomiting, back pain, cough, dyspnea

Special considerations:

- This medication may be taken with or without food.

- Patient should avoid alcohol consumption while on this medication.

(65)

Brand names: Flexeril, Amrix, Fexmid

Generic name: Cyclobenzaprine

Drug class: Skeletal muscle relaxant

- Treats musculoskeletal conditions such as muscle spasms and pain.

(66)

Brand name: Actonel

Generic name: Risedronate

Drug class: Calcium metabolism modifier, bisphosphonate

- Prevents osteoporosis in postmenopausal women.

(67)

Indication: Muscle spasms

Side effects: Drowsiness, dry mouth, dizziness, headache, nausea, palpitations, bad taste in mouth, indigestion, blurred vision, constipation

Special considerations:

- This medication should not be used concomitantly or within 14 days of discontinuing MAO inhibitors.
- This medication is not indicated for prolonged use (only 2–3 weeks).
- Patients on this medication should avoid use of alcohol.
- This medication can be taken with food to avoid stomach upset.

(66)

Indications: Osteoporosis treatment and prevention, Paget's disease

Side effects: Headache, pain, rash, diarrhea, abdominal pain, urinary tract infection, arthralgia, back pain, hypertension, peripheral edema, chest pain, cardiovascular disorder, angina, arrhythmia, depression, dizziness, insomnia, anxiety, pruritus, constipation, nausea, flatulence, belching, colitis, gastritis, prostatic hyperplasia, cystitis, nephrolithiasis, anemia, joint disorder, myalgia, neck pain, bone pain, weakness, neuralgia, leg cramps, myasthenia, cataract, dry eyes, pharyngitis, rhinitis, sinusitis, dyspnea, bronchitis, flu symptoms, neoplasm, hernia

Special considerations:

- This medication should be taken with plenty of water on an empty stomach about 30 minutes or more before the first drink or food of the day.
- Patients on this medication should ensure adequate intake of calcium and vitamin D.
- Patients should be instructed not to take this medication concurrently with aminoglycosides, NSAIDs, and antacids.

(67)

Brand name: Lasix

Generic name: Furosemide

Drug class: Loop diuretic

- Increases loss of water by elevating the rate of urination.

(68)

Brand names: Zofran, Zuplenz

Generic name: Ondansetron

Drug class: Antiemetic

- Prevents nausea and vomiting caused by chemotherapeutic agents.

(69)

Indications: Edema, hypertension

Side effects: Hyperuricemia, hypokalemia

Special considerations:

- This medication can lead to water and electrolyte depletion if taken in excessive amounts.
- Taking this medication with food will delay absorption.

(68)

Indications: Postoperative nausea and vomiting prophylaxis

Side effects: Headache, malaise/fatigue, diarrhea, dizziness, constipation, hypoxia, drowsiness, fever, anxiety, urinary retention, pruritus

Special consideration:

- This medication should be used only as a scheduled medication and not on an as-needed basis.

(69)

Brand names: Procardia XL, Adalat CC, Nifedical XL, Afeditab CR, Nifediac CC

Generic name: Nifedipine ER

Drug class: Calcium channel blocker

- Decreases blood pressure.

(70)

Brand names: Motrin, Advil, NeoProfen, Caldolor

Generic name: Ibuprofen

Drug class: NSAID

- Reduces fever (antipyretic), reduces inflammation (anti-inflammatory), and relieves pain (analgesic).

(71)

Indications: Angina, hypertension

Side effects: Peripheral edema, dizziness, flushing, headache, heartburn, nausea, muscle cramps, mood change, nervousness, cough, dyspnea, palpitations, wheezing, hypotension, constipation, chest pain

Special considerations:

- Patients who are lactose intolerant should not take the extended-release form of this medication because it contains lactose.

- Technicians should be aware that the immediate-acting (regular) form of this medication is not indicated for hypertension.

(70)

Indications: Pain, inflammation, fever

Side effects: Nausea, vomiting, headache, heartburn

Special considerations:

- Prolonged use of NSAIDs may increase risk of serious cardiovascular thrombotic events, myocardial infarction, and stroke.

- This medication can be taken with food, milk, or antacid to avoid stomach upset.

- Patients should be aware that overuse of NSAIDs can lead to serious GI adverse events including bleeding, ulceration, and perforation of the stomach or intestines.

(71)

Brand name: Folvite

Generic name: Folic acid

Drug class: Vitamin supplement (B_9)

- Water-soluble vitamin naturally found in leafy vegetables, fruits, beans, meat, orange juice, and tomato juice.

(72)

Brand names: Soma, Vanadom

Generic name: Carisoprodol

Drug class: Skeletal muscle relaxant

- Treats musculoskeletal conditions such as muscle spasms and pain.

(73)

Indication: Prevents and treats folate deficiency and other associated complications

Side effects: Allergic reaction, bronchospasm, flushing, malaise, pruritus, rash

Special consideration:

- Folic acid requirement is increased during pregnancy because deficiency may result in fetal harm.

(72)

Indication: Musculoskeletal conditions

Side effects: Drowsiness, dizziness, headache

Special considerations:

- This medication may lead to sedation.
- Patients should use caution with driving/operating machinery.

(73)

Brand name: Allegra D

Generic name: Fexofenadine/pseudoephedrine

Drug class: Antihistamine and decongestant combination

- Antihistamines counteract the effects of histamine, which is released in response to allergic reactions and produces an inflammatory response.

- Decongestants relieve nasal congestion.

(74)

Brand name: Ditropan XL

Generic name: Oxybutynin chloride ER

Drug class: Antispasmodic agent

- Prevents spasms of smooth muscles.

(75)

Indication: Seasonal allergic rhinitis with nasal congestion

Side effects: Headache, drowsiness, fatigue

Special considerations:

- This medication is contraindicated in premature newborns and neonates, and nursing women.

- Taking this medication with fruit juice may decrease its efficacy.

(74)

Indications: Symptoms of bladder instability, overactive bladder

Side effects: Dry mouth, constipation, somnolence, asthenia, dizziness, headache, blurred vision, dry eyes, diarrhea, nausea, pain, rhinitis

Special consideration:

- The patient should be aware that this medication should be discontinued if angioedema develops.

(75)

Brand name: Zantac

Generic name: Ranitidine HCl

Drug class: Histamine H_2 receptor antagonist

- Helps decrease stomach acid.

(76)

Brand name: Benicar

Generic name: Olmesartan

Drug class: Angiotensin receptor blocker (ARB)

- Notice the suffix *-sartan*, which distinguishes ARBs from other drug classes.

(77)

Indications: Gastroesophageal reflux disease (GERD), peptic ulcer disease, erosive esophagitis

Side effects: Headache, dizziness, agitation, confusion, constipation, diarrhea, nausea, abdominal pain, vomiting, alopecia, hypersensitivity reaction

Special consideration:

- This medication should not be taken by women who are breastfeeding.

(76)

Indication: Hypertension

Side effects: Dizziness, headache, hyperglycemia, diarrhea, back pain, hematuria, bronchitis, pharyngitis, rhinitis, sinusitis

Special consideration:

- Efficacy may be decreased with use of NSAIDs.

(77)

Brand names: Cipro, Proquin

Generic name: Ciprofloxacin HCl

Drug class: Fluoroquinolone antibiotic

- Treats both gram-negative and gram-positive bacteria.

- Notice the suffix *-oxacin,* which distinguishes fluoroquinolones from other drug classes.

(78)

Brand names: Adoxa, Doryx, Doxy-100, Monodox, Oracea, Periostat, Vibramycin, Vibra-tabs

Generic name: Doxycycline

Drug class: Tetracycline antibiotic

- Inhibits protein synthesis of susceptible bacteria.

(79)

Indications: Acute sinusitis, chronic bacterial prostatitis, infectious diarrhea, inhalational anthrax, lower respiratory tract infections, nosocomial pneumonia, urinary tract infection (UTI)

Side effects: Nausea, abdominal pain, diarrhea, vomiting, headache, rash, restlessness

Special considerations:

- This medication should be avoided in patients with a history of myasthenia gravis.

- This medication should not be taken with dairy products or calcium-fortified juices; antacids and vitamin or mineral supplements should be avoided within 6 hours before or 2 hours after taking this medication.

(78)

Indication: Infections caused by susceptible gram-positive and gram-negative organisms

Side effects: Intracranial hypertension, photosensitivity, rash, brown/black discoloration of thyroid gland, anorexia, diarrhea, enterocolitis, vomiting, dysphagia

Special considerations:

- Medications that end in the suffix *-cycline* are tetracycline-derivative antibiotics.

- Tetracycline can cause permanent discoloration (brown staining) in children under 8 years of age.

(79)

Brand names: Catapres, Duraclon, Jenloga, Kapvay, Nexiclon

Generic name: Clonidine

Drug class: Alpha$_2$ agonist

- Activates the alpha$_2$ receptor and exhibits sedative, analgesic, muscle relaxant, and anxiolytic effects.

(80)

Brand names: Klor-Con, K-Dur, Slow K, Kaon Cl 10, K10, Klotrix, K-Tab, Micro-K, K8

Generic name: Potassium chloride ER

Drug class: Electrolyte supplement

- Corrects electrolyte levels.

(81)

Indication: Hypertension

Side effects: Dry mouth, headache, fatigue, drowsiness, dizziness, nausea, vomiting

Special considerations:

- This medication has a black box warning stating that it is not recommended for use in obstetric postpartum or perioperative pain management.

- This medication should not be discontinued abruptly due to the risk of rebound hypertension.

- Patients should avoid the use of alcohol while on this medication.

(80)

Indications: Potassium supplementation, hypokalemia

Side effects: Arrhythmias, bleeding, diarrhea, dyspepsia, hyperkalemia, nausea, rash, vomiting

Special considerations:

- This medication is contraindicated with hyperkalemic patients.

- The injectable form of this medication cannot be given to patients via IV push/bolus, IM, or SC. This medication must be diluted before being infused so that the patient does not receive too much of it too quickly.

(81)

Brand names: Buprenex, Suboxone, Subutex

Generic name: Buprenorphine

Drug class: Opioid analgesic

- The injection formulation is used to manage moderate to severe pain. However, the tablet form is used for treating opioid dependence.

(82)

Brand name: Mobic

Generic name: Meloxicam

Drug class: NSAID

- Treats musculoskeletal conditions such as muscle spasms and pain.

(83)

Indication: Opioid withdrawal

Side effects: Sedation, hypotension, respiratory depression, dizziness, headache, vomiting, nausea, miosis, vertigo

Special considerations:

- The injection form of this medication is Schedule V, while the tablet form is Schedule III.

- This medication should not be taken with alcohol.

(82)

Indications: Rheumatoid arthritis, osteoarthritis

Side effects: Indigestion, upper respiratory infection, headache, diarrhea, nausea, abdominal pain, edema, anemia, dizziness, constipation, vomiting

Special considerations:

- This medication has a black box warning stating that prolonged use may increase the risk of possibly fatal serious cardiovascular thrombotic events, myocardial infarction (MI), and stroke, especially in patients with risk factors or existing cardiovascular disease.

- Patients should be aware that overuse of NSAIDs can lead to serious GI adverse events including bleeding, ulceration, and perforation of the stomach or intestines.

(83)

Brand name: Altace

Generic name: Ramipril

Drug class: Angiotensin-converting enzyme (ACE) inhibitor or blocker

- Decreases blood pressure and dilates blood vessels.

(84)

Brand names: Adipex, Ionamin, Suprenza

Generic name: Phentermine

Drug class: Amphetamine, CNS stimulant, anorexiant

- Suppresses appetite to treat obesity.

(85)

Indications: Hypertension, congestive heart failure (CHF) post-myocardial infarction (MI), MI/stroke risk

Side effects: Cough, hypotension, hyperkalemia, dizziness, fatigue, nausea, vomiting

Special considerations:

- This medication should not be taken by patients who are pregnant.

- Alert the pharmacist if a patient on an ACE inhibitor attempts to buy cough medication or complains of a cough. The cessation of the treatment is the only effective treatment for the ACE inhibitor-related cough.

(84)

Indication: Obesity

Side effects: Hypertension, palpitations, tachycardia, blurred vision, chills, dysphoric mood, dysuria, headache, insomnia, nervousness, restlessness, tremor

Special considerations:

- This medication is a Schedule IV habit-forming drug.

- This medication should be avoided by patients who have taken MAOIs within 14 days before initiation of therapy and patients who are on other CNS stimulants.

(85)

Brand name: Vasotec

Generic name: Enalapril

Drug class: Angiotensin-converting enzyme (ACE) inhibitor or blocker

- Decreases blood pressure and dilates blood vessels.

(86)

Brand name: Aldactone

Generic name: Spironolactone

Drug class: Potassium-sparing diuretic, aldosterone antagonist

- Treats fluid retention while sparing the loss of potassium.

(87)

Indications: Mild to severe hypertension, congestive heart failure (CHF), post-myocardial infarction (MI)

Side effects: Cough, hypotension, chest pain, syncope, orthostatic hypotension, headache, dizziness, fatigue, rash, bronchitis, cough, dyspnea

Special considerations:

- This medication should not be taken concurrently with diuretics, NSAIDs, and allopurinol.

- Patients should limit salt substitutes and a potassium-rich diet while on this medication.

(86)

Indications: Hyperaldosteronism, edema, hypertension, hypokalemia

Side effects: Drowsiness, lethargy, headache, mental confusion, rash

Special considerations:

- This medication has a black box warning pertaining to off-label uses due to its tumorigen nature.

- This medication should not be used concurrently with potassium-sparing diuretics or ACE inhibitors.

(87)

Brand name: Restoril

Generic name: Temazepam

Drug class: Benzodiazepine, hypnotic/sedative

- Treats anxiety and exhibits sedative effects.

(88)

Brand names: Desyrel, Oleptro

Generic name: Trazodone HCl

Drug class: Antidepressant

- Treats depression.

(89)

Indication: Insomnia

Side effects: Confusion, diarrhea, dizziness, drowsiness, euphoria, hangover, lethargy, vertigo, weakness

Special considerations:

- This medication may alter the patient's ability to perform hazardous tasks.

- Patients should avoid the use of alcohol while on this medication.

(88)

Indication: Depression

Side effects: Blurred vision, dizziness, drowsiness, dry mouth, fatigue, headache, nausea, vomiting

Special considerations:

- Patients should be aware that this medication has a black box warning stating the increased risk of suicidal thoughts and behavior in anyone under the age of 24.

- The drug should not be used in pediatric patients.

- This medication should not be taken at the same time as MAOIs; patients should allow at least 14 days before initiation of therapy.

- This medication is not recommended for young males because it may lead to prolonged and inappropriate erection.

(89)

Brand name: Actos

Generic name: Pioglitazone

Drug class: Oral antidiabetic, thiazolidinedione

- Improves glycemic control in adjunct to diet and exercise.

(90)

Brand name: Levemir

Generic name: Insulin Detemir

Drug class: Antidiabetic, insulin intermediate—long acting

- Controls hyperglycemia.

(91)

Indication: Type 2 diabetes mellitus (non-insulin-dependent diabetes)

Side effects: Edema, upper respiratory tract infection, heart failure, headache, fatigue, tooth disorders, anemia, myalgia, sinusitis, pharyngitis

Special considerations:

- This medication can be taken with or without food.

- Patients may experience increased risk for fractures while on this medication.

(90)

Indications: Type 1 diabetes mellitus (insulin-dependent diabetes) and type 2 diabetes mellitus (non-insulin-dependent diabetes)

Side effects: Itching, swelling, hypokalemia, wheezing, trouble breathing, sweating, weight gain, mild headache, back pain, stomach pain, flu symptoms

Special considerations:

- Insulin Detemir cannot be mixed with another insulin.

- This medication is for subcutaneous use and should not be administered intravenously or intramuscularly.

(91)

Brand names: Voltaren, Cataflam, Cambia, Zipsor

Generic name: Diclofenac sodium SR

Drug class: NSAID

- Treats musculoskeletal conditions such as muscle spasms and pain.

(92)

Brand names: Deltasone, Orasone, Sterapred

Generic name: Prednisone oral

Drug class: Corticosteroid

- Reduces inflammation.

(93)

Indications: Rheumatoid arthritis, osteoarthritis, inflammation, joint pain

Side effects: Abdominal distention and flatulence, abdominal pain or cramps, constipation, diarrhea, dyspepsia, nausea, peptic ulcer/GI bleeding, edema, fluid retention, pruritus, rash, tinnitus, dizziness, headache

Special considerations:

- Prolonged use of NSAIDs may increase risk of serious cardiovascular thrombotic events, myocardial infarction, and stroke.

- This medication can be taken with food, milk, or antacid to avoid stomach upset.

- Patients should be aware that overuse of NSAIDs can lead to serious GI adverse events including bleeding, ulceration, and perforation of the stomach or intestines.

(92)

Indications: Allergies, asthma

Side effects: Adrenal suppression, psychosis, insomnia, vertigo, acne, osteoporosis, myopathy, delayed wound healing

Special consideration:

- Patients should be aware that this medication is not indicated for long-term treatment.

(93)

Brand names: Dyazide, Maxzide

Generic name: Triamterene/hydrochlorothiazide (HCTZ)

Drug class: Thiazide diuretic combination

- Treats fluid retention and hypertension.

(94)

Brand names: Aleve, Naprosyn, Anaprox, Midol Extended Relief, Naprox Sodium, Naprelan, Pamprin All Day

Generic name: Naproxen

Drug class: NSAID

- Treats musculoskeletal conditions such as muscle spasms and pain.

(95)

Indication: Hypertension

Side effects: Congestive heart failure, edema, hypotension, dizziness, fatigue, anorexia, epigastric distress, hypokalemia, phototoxicity

Special consideration:

- This medication should be avoided in patients who are hypersensitive to triamterene, HCTZ, or sulfonamides.

(94)

Indications: Fever and minor aches and pains, rheumatoid arthritis, osteoarthritis

Side effects: Abdominal pain, constipation, heartburn, nausea, headache, dizziness, drowsiness, HI bleeding, GI perforation, GI ulcers, diarrhea

Special considerations:

- Prolonged use of NSAIDs may increase risk of serious cardiovascular thrombotic events, myocardial infarction, and stroke.

- This medication can be taken with food, milk, or antacid to avoid stomach upset.

- Patients should be aware that overuse of NSAIDs can lead to serious GI adverse events including bleeding, ulceration, and perforation of the stomach or intestines.

(95)

Brand name: Diflucan

Generic name: Fluconazole

Drug class: Antifungal

- Notice the suffix -*conazole*, which distinguishes antifungals from other drug classes.

(96)

Brand name: Levaquin

Generic name: Levofloxacin

Drug class: Fluoroquinolone antibiotic

- Broad-spectrum antibiotic that promotes breakage of DNA strands in susceptible organisms.

- Notice the suffix -*oxacin,* which distinguishes fluoroquinolones from other drug classes.

(97)

Indications: Candidiasis and other infections caused by susceptible organisms

Side effects: Headache, seizure, dizziness, rash, nausea, vomiting, abdominal pain, diarrhea, dyspepsia, dyspnea

Special consideration:

- Patient should take all medication as prescribed.

(96)

Indication: Infections caused by susceptible gram-positive and gram-negative organisms

Side effects: Chest pain, edema, headache, insomnia, dizziness, fatigue, pain, rash, pruritus, nausea, diarrhea, constipation, abdominal pain, dyspepsia, vomiting, vaginitis, pharyngitis, dyspnea

Special considerations:

- This medication should be avoided in patients with a history of myasthenia gravis.

- This medication should not be taken by children under 18 years of age.

- Patients should be informed to not take this medication with dairy products or calcium-fortified juices; antacids and vitamin or mineral supplements should be avoided within 6 hours before or 2 hours after taking this medication.

(97)

Brand name: Xarelto

Generic name: Rivaroxaban

Drug class: Factor Xa inhibitor, anticoagulant

- Prevents formation of blood clots.

(98)

Brand names: Valium, Diastat

Generic name: Diazepam

Drug class: Benzodiazepine, anticonvulsant, skeletal muscle relaxant, antianxiety agent, anxiolytic

- Produces sedation, induces sleep, reduces anxiety (anxiolytic), reduces seizures (anticonvulsant), and relaxes muscles.
- Notice the suffix *-pam*, which distinguishes benzodiazepines from other drug classes.

(99)

Indications: Deep vein thrombosis prophylaxis, pulmonary embolism

Side effects: Muscle pain; itching; easy bruising; bleeding; headache; dizziness; weakness; urine that looks red, pink, or brown; bloody or tarry stools

Special considerations:

- Patients should be monitored for bleeding while on this medication.

- Doses equal to or larger than 15 mg must be taken with food.

(98)

Indications: Anxiety disorders, muscle spasms

Side effects: Ataxia, euphoria, incoordination, somnolence, rash, diarrhea

Special considerations:

- This is a Schedule IV habit-forming drug.

- The patient should not take this medication with alcohol.

(99)

Brand names: Cleocin, Clindesse, ClindaMax Vaginal

Generic name: Clindamycin

Drug class: Antibiotic

- Treats bacterial infections by susceptible organisms.

(100)

Brand name: Celebrex

Generic name: Celecoxib

Drug class: NSAID, COX-2 receptor blocker

- Nonsteroidal anti-inflammatory drugs (NSAIDs) have antipyretic (fever reducing), anti-inflammatory, and analgesic (pain-relieving) effects.

(101)

Indications: Serious bacterial infections, anthrax, amnionitis, bacterial vaginosis

Side effects: Abdominal pain, diarrhea, fungal overgrowth, rashes, nausea, vomiting, hypotension

Special considerations:

- This medication has a black box warning stating that it may result in mild diarrhea to fatal colitis, which may require colectomy.
- This medication should not be used over a long period of time.
- Patients should finish the full course of therapy unless otherwise instructed by their physician.

(100)

Indications: Osteoarthritis, rheumatoid arthritis, acute pain, primary dysmenorrhea

Side effects: Hypertension, headache, diarrhea, peripheral edema, fever, insomnia, dizziness, skin rash, dyspepsia, nausea, gastroesophageal reflux, abdominal pain, vomiting, flatulence, upper respiratory tract infection, cough, nasopharyngitis, sinusitis, dyspnea, pharyngitis, rhinitis

Special considerations:

- Patients should avoid taking sulfonamides, aspirin, and other NSAIDs while on this medication.
- Prolonged use of NSAIDs may increase risk of serious cardiovascular thrombotic events, myocardial infarction, and hypertension.
- Patients should be aware that overuse of NSAIDs can lead to serious GI adverse events including bleeding, ulceration, and perforation of the stomach or intestines.

(101)

Brand name: Tylenol #2

Generic name: Codeine/acetaminophen

Drug class: Narcotic, opioid analgesic, antipyretic

- Relieves pain and reduces fever.

(102)

Brand names: Nasonex, Asmanex, Twisthaler, Elocon

Generic name: Mometasone

Drug class: Corticosteroid, intranasal

- Reduces inflammation and mucus production.

(103)

Indication: Moderate to moderately severe pain relief

Side effects: Lightheadedness, dizziness, drowsiness or sedation, nausea, vomiting

Special considerations:

- This medication is a Schedule II habit-forming drug.

- The patient should not use this medication in combination with acetaminophen or other products containing acetaminophen in order to not exceed the maximum dose allowance of acetaminophen (doses that exceed 4 g of acetaminophen per day).

- The patient should not take this medication with alcohol.

(102)

Indication: Allergic and nonallergic nasal symptoms of rhinitis

Side effects: Headache, fatigue, depression, musculoskeletal pain, arthralgia, sinusitis, rhinitis, upper respiratory infection, pharyngitis, cough, viral infection, oral candidiasis, vomiting

Special considerations:

- Patients with recent nasal injury or surgery should avoid this medication.

- Hypoglycemic effects of antidiabetic agents may be decreased by corticosteroids.

(103)

Brand name: Lyrica

Generic name: Pregabalin

Drug class: Analgesic, anticonvulsant, antiepileptic

- Slows down impulses in the brain responsible for seizures and signals that result in pain.

(104)

Brand name: Novolog

Generic name: Insulin aspart

Drug class: Antidiabetic, insulin fast-acting

- Controls hyperglycemia.

(105)

Indications: Neuropathic pain associated with diabetes, fibromyalgia

Side effects: Peripheral edema, dizziness, somnolence, ataxia, headache, weight gain, dry mouth, tremor, blurred vision, diplopia, infection, accidental injury, chest pain, edema, neuropathy, fatigue, confusion, euphoria, speech disorder, attention disturbance, incoordination, amnesia, pain, impaired memory, vertigo, feeling abnormal, constipation, appetite increased, flatulence, vomiting, incontinence, thrombocytopenia, balance disorder, weakness, twitching, back pain, muscle spasm

Special consideration:

- This medication is a Schedule V habit-forming drug.

(104)

Indications: Type 1 diabetes mellitus (insulin-dependent diabetes) and type 2 diabetes mellitus (non-insulin-dependent diabetes)

Side effects: Itching skin rash, wheezing, trouble breathing, sweating, fast heart rate, swelling, hypokalemia

Special considerations:

- This medication is usually administered before a meal.

- This medication is for subcutaneous use and should not be administered intravenously or intramuscularly.

- It is important not to confuse this medication with other insulins.

(105)

Brand name: Zetia

Generic name: Ezetimibe

Drug class: Antilipemic

- Lowers high cholesterol.

(106)

Brand name: Premarin

Generic name: Conjugated estrogens

Drug class: Hormone replacement

- Major class of female hormones.

(107)

Indication: Hypercholesterolemia

Side effects: Upper respiratory tract infection, chest pain, headache, dizziness, fatigue, diarrhea, abdominal pain, myalgia, arthralgia, back pain, sinusitis, pharyngitis, cough

Special considerations:

- Patients should watch their dietary intake and exercise while taking this medication.

(106)

Indications: Menopausal moderate to severe vasomotor symptoms, hypogonadism, prostatic cancer, osteoporosis, abnormal uterine bleeding

Side effects: Headache, breast pain, abdominal pain, vaginal hemorrhage, back pain, nervousness, pruritus, flatulence, vaginitis, leucorrhea, weakness, leg cramps

Special considerations:

- This medication can be taken with food to reduce chances of gastrointestinal upset.
- This medication may increase chances of uterine cancer.

(107)

Brand names: Zyloprim, Aloprim

Generic name: Allopurinol

Drug class: Xanthine oxidase inhibitor, antigout

- Reduces production of uric acid.

(108)

Brand names: Pen VK, Veetids

Generic name: Penicillin V potassium

Drug class: Penicillin antibiotic

- Kills bacteria by interfering with their cell wall formation.

(109)

Indications: Primary or secondary gout, elevated uric acid levels in cancer patients

Side effects: Rash, nausea, vomiting, drowsiness, headache, muscle pain

Special considerations:

- Patients should drink 8 to 10 full glasses of water daily to prevent kidney stone formation.

- This medication should be discontinued at first sign of a rash.

(108)

Indication: Bacterial infections caused by susceptible organisms

Side effects: Anaphylaxis, anemia, candidiasis, diarrhea, headache, nausea, rash, vomiting

Special considerations:

- The patient should not take this medication if allergic to penicillins, cephalosporins, or carbapenems.

- The medication should be completed as prescribed.

- The medication should be taken with food to avoid gastrointestinal upset.

(109)

Brand name: Januvia

Generic name: Sitagliptin

Drug class: Antihyperglycemic, antidiabetic, dipeptidyl peptidase-4 inhibitor (DPP-4 inhibitor)

- Lowers blood glucose levels by stimulating the release of insulin and decreasing glucagon secretion.
- Improves glycemic control in adjunct to diet and exercise.

(110)

Brand name: Elavil

Generic name: Amitriptyline

Drug class: Tricyclic antidepressant (TCA)

- Treats depression.

(111)

Indication: Type 2 diabetes mellitus (non-insulin-dependent diabetes)

Side effects: Upper respiratory tract infection, nasopharyngitis, nausea, and headache

Special considerations:

- This medication is contraindicated in patients with type 1 diabetes.

- The patient's renal function should be monitored while on this medication.

(110)

Indications: Depression, chronic pain, migraine prophylaxis

Side effects: Anticholinergic effects, orthostatic hypotension, tachycardia, MI, stroke, heart block, arrhythmia, syncope, hypertension, palpitation, restlessness, dizziness, insomnia, sedation, fatigue, anxiety, impaired cognitive function, seizure, extrapyramidal symptoms, hallucinations, confusion, ataxia, headache, urticaria, alopecia, weight gain, nausea, vomiting, anorexia, stomatitis, blurred vision, mydriasis, numbness, tremor, weakness

Special considerations:

- This medication should not be used with monoamine oxidase inhibitors (MAOIs).

- Patients on this medication should avoid alcohol.

- This medication should not be stopped abruptly without physician recommendation.

(111)

Brand name: Xalatan

Generic name: Latanoprost

Drug class: Antiglaucoma, ophthalmic agent, prostaglandin

- Treats glaucoma by lowering pressure in the eye.

(112)

Brand name: Vyvanse

Generic name: Lisdexamfetamine

Drug class: CNS stimulant, ADHD agent

(113)

Indications: Open-angle glaucoma, ocular hypertension

Side effects: Ocular burning, stinging, discomfort, blurred vision, redness of the eye, eyelid darkening, dry eye, increased photosensitivity, flu-like symptoms

Special consideration:

- This medication should be refrigerated.

(112)

Indication: Attention deficit hyperactivity disorder (ADHD)

Side effects: Insomnia, headache, abdominal pain, decrease in appetite, irritability, dizziness, fever, somnolence, tic, vomiting, weight loss, nausea, dry mouth, rash

Special considerations:

- This is a Schedule II habit-forming drug.

- The patient should not take concurrently with monoamine oxidase inhibitors (MAOIs).

- Patients with hypertension, advanced arteriosclerosis, or other serious heart problems should avoid this medication.

(113)

Brand name: Niaspan

Generic name: Niacin

Drug class: Antilipemic, vitamin B_3

- Water-soluble vitamin.

(114)

Brand name: Dexilant

Generic name: Dexlansoprazole

Drug class: Proton pump inhibitor (PPI)

- Prevents acid buildup.

- Notice the suffix *-prazole*, which distinguishes PPIs from other drug classes.

(115)

Indications: Recurrent MI, coronary artery disease, hypertriglyceridemia, peripheral vascular disease and circulatory disorders, pellagra, dietary supplement

Side effects: Flushing, arrhythmias, arterial fibrillation, edema, flushing, hypotension, palpitation, tachycardia, chills, dizziness, headache, insomnia, migraine, nervousness, pain, dry skin, rash, gout, abdominal pain, diarrhea, flatulence, nausea, vomiting, peptic ulcers, jaundice, myalgia, weakness, dyspnea

Special considerations:

- Patients should be advised to avoid alcohol.

- This medication should be taken at bedtime with a low-fat snack.

- Patients should be aware that consuming over 2 grams of this medication per day can cause hepatotoxicity.

(114)

Indications: Gastroesophageal reflux disease (GERD), ulcers, heartburn

Side effects: Gas, nausea, vomiting, rash, hives, itching, difficulty breathing or swallowing, irregular heartbeat, excessive tiredness, dizziness, lightheadedness, muscle spasms, seizures, severe diarrhea, stomach pain, fever

Special considerations:

- The patient should not take this medication if hypersensitive to other proton pump inhibitors.

- PPIs increase the risk of fracturing wrists, hips, or spine.

- Serious side effects should be reported to the physician.

(115)

Brand names: Diabeta, Glynase, PresTab, Micronase

Generic name: Glyburide

Drug class: Antihyperglycemic, antidiabetic agent, sulfonylurea

- Stimulates insulin release while reducing glucose output from the liver.

(116)

Brand names: Zyprexa, Zydis

Generic name: Olanzapine

Drug class: Atypical antipsychotic

- Exhibits antagonistic effects on the dopamine and serotonin receptors.

(117)

Indication: Type 2 diabetes mellitus (non-insulin-dependent diabetes)

Side effects: Vasculitis, headache, dizziness, erythema, pruritus, purpura, rash, urticaria, photosensitivity, hypoglycemia, hyponatremia, nausea, heartburn, constipation, diarrhea, anorexia, nocturia, hepatitis, arthralgia, myalgia, blurred vision

Special considerations:

- Patients should take this medication with meals at the same time daily.

- Patients should be aware that symptoms of hypoglycemia include palpitations, sweaty palms, and lightheadedness.

(116)

Indications: Schizophrenia, bipolar mania

Side effects: Somnolence, extrapyramidal symptoms, insomnia, dizziness, dyspepsia, constipation, weight gain, dry mouth, weakness, postural hypotension, tachycardia, peripheral edema, chest pain, personality changes, speech disorder, fever, bruising, nausea, appetite increase, vomiting, incontinence, tremor, back pain, rhinitis, cough, dyspnea

Special consideration:

- This medication may be taken without consideration of food.

(117)

Brand name: Detrol

Generic name: Tolterodine

Drug class: Anticholinergic agent, muscarinic antagonist

- Treats urinary bladder disease.

(118)

Brand name: Pepcid

Generic name: Famotidine

Drug class: Histamine H_2 receptor antagonist

- Helps decrease stomach acid.

(119)

Indication: Overactive bladder

Side effects: Dry mouth, chest pain, headache, somnolence, fatigue, dizziness, anxiety, dry skin, abdominal pain, constipation, dyspepsia, diarrhea, weight gain, dysuria, arthralgia, blurred vision, drowsiness, dry eyes, bronchitis, flulike syndrome

Special consideration:

- Patients should be advised not to operate machinery or drive while on this medication because it may impair physical or mental abilities.

(118)

Indications: Duodenal ulcer, gastroesophageal reflux disease (GERD), benign gastric ulcer

Side effects: Agitation, vomiting, headache, dizziness, diarrhea, constipation, abdominal discomfort, acne, alopecia, anaphylaxis, anorexia, anxiety, arrhythmia, arthralgia, bradycardia, bronchospasm, confusion, depression, fatigue, fever, flushing, insomnia, nausea, somnolence

Special consideration:

- This medication should not be taken by women who are breastfeeding.

(119)

Brand name: Lantus

Generic name: Insulin glargine

Drug class: Antidiabetic, long-acting insulin (up to 24 hrs)

- Controls hyperglycemia.

(120)

Brand name: Armour Thyroid

Generic name: Thyroid

Drug class: Thyroid hormone

- Treats underactive thyroid.

(121)

Indications: Type 1 diabetes mellitus (insulin-dependent diabetes), type 2 diabetes mellitus (non-insulin-dependent diabetes)

Side effects: Itching, swelling, rash, hives, wheezing, shortness of breath, sweating, hoarseness, weakness, muscle cramps, abnormal heartbeat

Special considerations:

- Insulin glargine cannot be mixed with another insulin.

- This medication may cause an increase in pain at injection site.

- Patients should limit alcohol consumption while on this medication because it can increase the risk of hypoglycemia.

(120)

Indications: Hypothyroidism, goiter

Side effects: Weight loss, tremor, headache, nausea, vomiting, diarrhea, stomach cramps, hyperactivity, anxiety, irritability, difficulty falling asleep or staying asleep, flushing, increase in appetite, fever, muscle weakness, temporary hair loss

Special considerations:

- This medication should not be used for treatment of obesity or for weight loss.

- This medication should be taken in the morning on an empty stomach.

(121)

Brand name: Zyrtec

Generic name: Cetirizine hydrochloride

Drug class: Antihistamine (2nd generation)

- Blocks the release of histamines.

(122)

Brand name: Lunesta

Generic name: Eszopiclone

Drug class: Sedative, hypnotic

- Treats insomnia.

(123)

Indications: Hay fever, perennial and seasonal allergies, urticaria

Side effects: Drowsiness, headache, somnolence, insomnia, dizziness, excessive tiredness, dry mouth, stomach pain, diarrhea, nausea, vomiting

Special considerations:

- The patient should not take this medication with alcohol.

- This medication should not be taken simultaneously with CNS depressants and anticholinergics.

(122)

Indication: Insomnia

Side effects: Dizziness, headache, unpleasant taste, chest pain, peripheral edema, somnolence, pain, nervousness, anxiety, depression, diarrhea, drowsiness, dry mouth, hallucinations, vomiting, rash, pruritus, decreased libido, dysmenorrhea, neuralgia, infection

Special considerations:

- This medication is a Schedule IV controlled substance.

- Patients on this medication should avoid use of alcohol and other CNS depressants.

- Patients should not take this medication after a heavy meal because it may reduce the onset of action.

(123)

Brand name: Zovirax

Generic name: Acyclovir

Drug class: Antiviral

- Treats viral infection.

(124)

Brand name: Colcrys

Generic name: Colchicine

Drug class: Antigout

- Reduces uric acid deposition on the joints.

(125)

Indications: Genital herpes simplex virus (HSV), cold sores, herpes zoster (shingles), varicella-zoster (chickenpox)

Side effects: Malaise, headache, nausea, vomiting, diarrhea, hives, itching, rash, phlebitis, mild pain, burning, stinging, pruritus, itching, abdominal pain

Special considerations:

- This medication interacts with the herpes zoster vaccine.
- Patients should avoid intercourse during herpes outbreaks.
- Patients should stay well hydrated during herpes outbreaks.

(124)

Indication: Treatment and prevention of acute gouty arthritis attacks

Side effects: Nausea, vomiting, diarrhea, abdominal pain, alopecia, anorexia

Special considerations:

- Tablets are light sensitive.
- Patients should avoid alcohol while on this medication.

(125)

Brand name: Lopid

Generic name: Gemfibrozil

Drug class: Antilipemic, fibric acid derivative

- Lowers the amount of cholesterol and triglycerides in the blood.

(126)

Brand names: Robitussin, Diabetic Tussin, Mucinex

Generic name: Guaifenesin

Drug class: Expectorant

- Makes coughs more productive by loosening phlegm and bronchial secretions.

(127)

Indications: Hypertriglyceridemia, hyperlipidemia

Side effects: Dyspepsia, fatigue, vertigo, headache, eczema, rash, abdominal pain, diarrhea, nausea/vomiting, constipation

Special considerations:

- This medication should be taken 30 minutes before breakfast and dinner.
- This medication is contraindicated in patients with severe liver/renal dysfunction, primary biliary cirrhosis, and pre-existing gallbladder disease.
- Patients should discontinue medication and immediately report to the physician signs of urine discoloration (brown) or muscle pain.
- This medication may increase risk of gallstones.

(126)

Indication: Productive cough

Side effects: Dizziness, drowsiness, headache, rash, decrease in uric acid, nausea, vomiting, stomach pain

Special considerations:

- This medication should not be used for persistent or chronic cough or coughs associated with excessive phlegm release.
- This medication should be taken with plenty of water.

(127)

Brand names: Glucotrol, Glucotrol XL

Generic name: Glipizide

Drug class: Antidiabetic, sulfonylurea

- Controls blood sugar by stimulating release of insulin by beta cells.

(128)

Brand name: Avapro

Generic name: Irbesartan

Drug class: Angiotensin receptor blocker (ARB)

- Notice the suffix *-sartan*, which distinguishes ARBs from other drug classes.

(129)

Indication: Type 2 diabetes mellitus (non-insulin-dependent diabetes)

Side effects: Hypoglycemia, nausea, diarrhea, constipation, gastralgia, erythema, urticaria, pruritus, eczema, leukopenia, agranulocytosis, thrombocytopenia, hemolytic anemia, aplastic anemia, pancytopenia, hyponatremia, dizziness, drowsiness, headache

Special considerations:

- Oral hypoglycemics are associated with improved positive outcome in cardiovascular treatment.

- Patients should diet and exercise while on this medication.

(128)

Indications: Hypertension, diabetic nephropathy

Side effects: Hyperkalemia in patients with diabetic nephropathy, orthostatic hypotension, fatigue, dizziness, diarrhea, dyspepsia, upper respiratory infection, cough, musculoskeletal pain, urticaria, rhabdomyolysis

Special considerations:

- Patients should not use this medication if pregnant.

- Patients should avoid taking this medication with NSAIDs, potassium-sparing diuretics, and salt substitutes.

(129)

Brand name: Reglan

Generic name: Metoclopramide

Drug class: Antiemetic, gastrointestinal agent

- Treats nausea and vomiting.

(130)

Brand names: Dramamine, Antivert

Generic name: Meclizine

Drug class: Antihistamine, antiemetic, antivertigo

- Prevents nausea and vomiting.

(131)

Indications: GERD, emesis, diabetic gastroparesis, persistent heartburn

Side effects: Drowsiness, fatigue, restlessness, dystonic reactions, trouble sleeping, agitation, headache, diarrhea

Special considerations:

- This medication should be taken 30 minutes before a meal.

- Patients on this medication should avoid consumption of alcohol.

- This medication is associated with extrapyramidal symptoms and depression.

(130)

Indications: Motion sickness, vertigo

Side effects: Drowsiness, cough, difficulty swallowing, dizziness, fast heartbeat, hives, itching, swelling, shortness of breath, skin rash, tightness in chest, unusual tiredness or weakness

Special consideration:

- This medication should not be taken with alcohol.

(131)

Brand name: Flagyl

Generic name: Metronidazole

Drug class:

- Amebicide, antibiotic, antiprotozoal, nitroimidazole

(132)

Brand name: Caltrate

Generic name: Calcium carbonate and vitamin D_3

Drug class: Calcium supplement

- Calcium strengthens bones and is needed for the heart, muscles, and nerves to function properly. Vitamin D helps the body absorb calcium.

(133)

Indication: Infections caused by susceptible anaerobic bacterial and protozoal organisms

Side effects: Convulsive seizures, encephalopathy, aseptic meningitis, optic and peripheral neuropathy, headache, syncope, dizziness, vertigo, incoordination, ataxia, confusion, dysarthria, irritability, depression, weakness, insomnia, rash, pruritus

Special considerations:

- Patients should complete all medications as prescribed by the physician.

- Patients should avoid alcohol consumption while on this medication and 2 days after.

- This medication may discolor urine to a reddish-brown color.

(132)

Indications: Treatment or prevention of calcium deficiency and osteoporosis

Side effects: Rash, hives, itching, difficulty breathing, tightness in chest, swelling, loss of appetite, nausea, constipation, vomiting

Special consideration:

- This medication should not be used in patients with high blood calcium or high blood vitamin D levels.

(133)

Brand name: AndroGel

Generic name: Testosterone

Drug class: Androgen

- Androgen replacement therapy.

(134)

Brand name: Requip

Generic name: Ropinirole

Drug class: Anti-Parkinson's agent, dopamine agonist

- Acts on dopamine receptors and treats the symptoms of Parkinson's disease.

(135)

Indications: Delayed male puberty, hypogonadism, inoperable metastatic female breast cancer

Side effects: Deep venous thrombosis, edema, hypertension, vasodilation, aggressive behavior, amnesia, anxiety, dizziness, excitation, headache, malaise, mental depression, nervousness, seizure, sleep apnea, sleeplessness, acne, alopecia, dry skin, hirsutism, pruritus, rash, breast soreness, growth acceleration, gynecomastia, hypercholesterolemia, hyperlipidemia, nausea, vomiting, weight gain, anemia, bleeding

Special considerations:

- Women who are pregnant should avoid touching this medication or having skin-to-skin contact in areas where testosterone has been applied.

(134)

Indications: Parkinson's disease, moderate to severe restless legs syndrome

Side effects: Syncope, somnolence, dizziness, fatigue, nausea, vomiting, viral infection, leg edema, orthostatic hypotension, hypertension, chest pain, flushing, palpitation, peripheral ischemia, hypotension, tachycardia, pain, confusion, hallucinations, anxiety, amnesia, malaise, vertigo, yawning, insomnia, neuralgia, constipation, dyspepsia, abdominal pain, dry mouth, diarrhea, anorexia, flatulence, dysphagia, salivation increase, urinary tract infection, impotence, anemia, arthralgia, weakness, tremor, arthritis, rhinitis, dyspnea, nasal congestion

Special considerations:

- Patients who develop sudden daytime "sleep attacks" should discontinue this medication.

- Patients should avoid consumption of alcohol or other sedative drugs while on this medication.

(135)

Brand names: Pazeo, Patanol, Pataday

Generic name: Olopatadine hydrochloride

Drug class: Antihistamine, ophthalmic agent

- Blocks the release of histamines.

(136)

Brand names: Avelox, Vigamox, Avelox IV

Generic name: Moxifloxacin hydrochloride

Drug class: Fluoroquinolone antibiotic, ophthalmic agent

- Treats both gram-negative and gram-positive bacteria.

(137)

Indication: Treatment of allergic conjunctivitis

Side effects: Cold syndrome, headache, pharyngitis, nausea, back pain, weakness, blurred vision, burning, conjunctivitis, dry eyes, eye pain, cough, rhinitis, flulike syndrome

Special consideration:

- Patients who wear contact lenses should remove contact lenses before instilling the medication and wait 10 minutes before reinserting.

(136)

Indications: Mild to moderate pneumonia, bronchitis, sinusitis, skin infections, abdominal bacterial infections, bacterial conjunctivitis (ophthalmic agent)

Side effects: Dizziness, nausea, diarrhea, palpitation, tachycardia, vasodilation, anxiety, headache, insomnia, malaise, nervousness, pain, somnolence, vertigo, pruritus, rash, urticaria, abdominal pain

Special considerations:

- This medication should be discontinued in patients who experience significant CNS adverse effects or tendon inflammation and/or pain.
- Fluoroquinolones are associated with serious hypoglycemic episodes.
- This medication should be taken 8 hours after or 4 hours before administration of multiple vitamins, antacids, or other medications containing magnesium, aluminum, iron, or zinc.

(137)

Brand name: Focalin

Generic name: Dexmethylphenidate hydrochloride

Drug class: Central nervous system stimulant

- Excites the nervous system.

(138)

Brand name: Bentyl

Generic name: Dicyclomine hydrochloride

Drug class: Anticholinergic

- Reduces spasms of the gastrointestinal tract.

(139)

Indication: Treatment of attention deficit hyperactivity disorder (ADHD)

Side effects: Stomach pain, loss of appetite, dizziness, nausea, vomiting, heartburn, weight loss, dry mouth, difficulty falling asleep, dizziness, drowsiness, nervousness, headache

Special considerations:

- This is a Schedule II habit-forming drug.

- The patient should not take concurrently with monoamine oxidase inhibitors (MAOIs).

(138)

Indication: Irritable bowel syndrome (IBS)

Side effects: Dry mouth, upset stomach, vomiting, constipation, stomach pain, gas, loss of appetite, dizziness, tingling, headache, drowsiness, weakness, blurred vision, double vision, difficulty urinating

Special considerations:

- Patients should avoid alcohol consumption while on this medication.

- Breastfeeding patients should not take this medication.

(139)

Brand name: Zebeta

Generic name: Bisoprolol

Drug class: Beta blocker, beta$_1$ selective blocker

- Relaxes blood vessels and slows heart rate.

- Notice the suffix *-olol*, which distinguishes beta blockers from other drug classes.

(140)

Brand name: Strattera

Generic name: Atomoxetine hydrochloride

Drug class: Norepinephrine reuptake inhibitor, nonstimulant

- Increases the levels of norepinephrine.

(141)

Indication: Hypertension

Side effects: Tiredness, vomiting, diarrhea, muscle aches, runny nose

Special considerations:

- Patients should avoid alcohol consumption while on this medication.

- Patients should not discontinue this medication abruptly.

(140)

Indication: Treatment of attention deficit hyperactivity disorder (ADHD)

Side effects: Heartburn, nausea, vomiting, loss of appetite, weight loss, constipation, stomach pain, gas, dry mouth, excessive tiredness, dizziness, headache, mood swings, decreased sex drive, difficulty urinating, painful or irregular menstrual periods, muscle pain, sweating, hot flashes, unusual dreams, burning or tingling sensation

Special considerations:

- The patient should not take concurrently with monoamine oxidase inhibitors (MAOIs).

- Patients should avoid alcohol consumption while on this medication.

- This medication may cause orthostatic hypotension.

(141)

Brand names: Adipex P, Ionamin

Generic name: Phentermine hydrochloride

Drug class: CNS stimulant, sympathomimetic, appetite suppressant

- Weight management for obese patients.

(142)

Brand name: Accupril

Generic name: Quinapril

Drug class: Angiotensin-converting enzyme (ACE) inhibitor

- Decreases blood pressure and dilates blood vessels.

(143)

Indication: Obesity management

Side effects: Hypertension, palpitation, cardiac vascular disease, tachycardia, dizziness, dysphoria, euphoria, headache, insomnia, overstimulation, psychosis, restlessness, change in libido, constipation, diarrhea, unpleasant taste, dry mouth, impotence, tremor

Special considerations:

- This is a Schedule IV habit-forming drug.

- This medication should be taken in the morning before breakfast or 1 to 2 hours after breakfast.

(142)

Indications: Hypertension, congestive heart failure

Side effects: Hypotension, chest pain, dizziness, headache, fatigue, rash, hyperkalemia, vomiting, nausea, myalgia, back pain, cough, dyspnea

Special considerations:

- This medication should not be used in the second or third trimesters of pregnancy due to potential harm and death to the developing fetus.

- Alert pharmacist if a patient on an ACE inhibitor attempts to buy cough medication or complains of a cough. The cessation of the treatment is the only effective treatment for the ACE inhibitor-related cough.

(143)

Brand names: Viagra, Revatio

Generic name: Sildenafil

Drug class: Phosphodiesterase-5 enzyme (PDE) inhibitor

- Relaxes blood vessels in the lungs, thereby increasing blood flow.

(144)

Brand name: Tamiflu

Generic name: Oseltamivir

Drug class: Antiviral

- Blocks the action of types A and B influenza virus.

(145)

Indications: Erectile dysfunction, pulmonary arterial hypertension

Side effects: Flushing, diarrhea, myalgia, headache, dyspepsia, insomnia, dizziness, erythema, rash, gastritis, urinary tract infection, abnormal vision, nasal congestion, rhinitis, sinusitis

Special considerations:

- This medication should not be taken concurrently with grapefruit juice.

- This medication should not be used concurrently with nitrates in any form.

(144)

Indication: Treatment and prophylaxis against influenza A or B

Side effects: Vomiting, nausea, abdominal pain, allergy, anaphylactic reaction, arrhythmia, confusion, dermatitis, eczema, rash, seizure, Stevens-Johnson syndrome

Special consideration:

- This medication can be taken with or without food.

(145)

Brand names: Rheumatrex, Trexall

Generic name: Methotrexate

Drug class: Antineoplastic, antimetabolite, disease-modifying antirheumatic

- Slows the growth of cells and the activity of the immune system.

(146)

Brand name: Pradaxa

Generic name: Dabigatran

Drug class: Anticoagulant, direct thrombin inhibitor

- Prevents formation of blood clots

(147)

Indications: Psoriasis, rheumatoid arthritis, cancer

Side effects: Reddening of skin, hyperuricemia, ulcerative stomatitis, gingivitis, nausea, vomiting, diarrhea, anorexia, dizziness, drowsiness, headache, swollen gums, decreased appetite, hair loss, blurred vision, seizures, confusion, weakness, loss of consciousness

Special considerations:

- This medication is contraindicated in pregnancy.

- This medication should not be used concurrently with NSAIDs.

(146)

Indications: Reduce the risk of stroke and blood clots (deep venous thrombosis, pulmonary embolism) in people diagnosed with atrial fibrillation

Side effects: Stomach pain, upset stomach, heartburn, nausea, unusual bruising or bleeding, pink or brown urine, red or black tarry stools, coughing up blood, gum bleeding, frequent nosebleeds, heavy menstrual bleeding, joint pain, headache, dizziness, weakness, hives, rash, itching, chest pain, difficulty breathing, swelling

Special considerations:

- This medication is contraindicated in pregnancy.

- Patients should report unusual bleeding or bruising and discoloration of urine or feces to their doctor.

(147)

Brand names: Uceris, Entocort EC

Generic name: Budesonide

Drug class: Corticosteroid

- Decreases inflammation in the digestive tract.

(148)

Brand name: Cardura

Generic name: Doxazosin

Drug class: Alpha^1-adrenergic blocker, antihypertensive

- Relaxes veins and arteries so that blood can flow easily.

(149)

Indication: Treatment of Crohn's disease

Side effects: Headache, nausea, respiratory infection, rhinitis, chest pain, edema, flushing, hypertension, palpitation, syncope, tachycardia, dizziness, fatigue, fever, insomnia, migraine, nervousness, pain, vertigo, acne, alopecia, bruising, dry mouth, vomiting, weight gain

Special considerations:

- Patients should avoid eating grapefruit and drinking grapefruit juice while on this medication.

- This medication is contraindicated in pregnancy.

(148)

Indications: Hypertension, urinary outflow obstruction, obstructive symptoms in patients with benign prostatic hyperplasia (BPH)

Side effects: Light-headedness, stomach pain, chest pain, trouble breathing

Special consideration:

- This medication may cause orthostatic hypotension after first dose or dose increase.

(149)

Brand name: Pristiq

Generic name: Desvenlafaxine

Drug class: Antidepressant, serotonin–norepinephrine reuptake inhibitor (SNRI)

- Treats depression by increasing the supply of serotonin and norepinephrine in the brain.

(150)

Brand name: Humalog

Generic name: Insulin lispro

Drug class: Antidiabetic, rapid-acting insulin

- Controls hyperglycemia.

(151)

Indication: Depression

Side effects: Constipation, loss of appetite, dry mouth, dizziness, extreme tiredness, unusual dreams, yawning, sweating, shaking, pain, burning, numbness, tingling, mydriasis, change in libido, difficulty urinating

Special considerations:

- This medication should not be taken concurrently with monoamine oxidase inhibitors (MAOIs).

- The patient should wait 14 days before initiating therapy after being on an MAOI or 7 days before taking an MAOI after stopping this medication.

- The patient should not discontinue this medication abruptly.

- Patients should be aware that this medication should not be taken with alcohol.

- This medication may cause drowsiness. Patients should not operate heavy machinery until they know how this medication will affect them.

(150)

Indication: Type 1 diabetes mellitus (insulin-dependent diabetes) and type 2 diabetes mellitus (non-insulin-dependent diabetes)

Side effects: Itching, rash, wheezing, shortness of breath, tachycardia, sweating, hypoglycemia, hypokalemia, weight gain, constipation

Special considerations:

- An increased risk of hypoglycemia is associated with insulin lispro if meal ingestion or absorption is delayed.

- This medication should be taken immediately before meals.

(151)

Brand name: Biaxin

Generic name: Clarithromycin

Drug class: Macrolide antibiotic

- Stops bacterial growth by interfering with its ability to make protein.

- Notice the suffix -*romycin*, which distinguishes macrolide antibiotics from other drug classes.

(152)

Brand name: Buspar

Generic name: Buspirone

Drug class: Antianxiety, anxiolytic

- Decreases action and amount of serotonin in the brain.

(153)

Indications: Mild to moderate upper respiratory bacterial infections, acute sinusitis, acute otitis media, pharyngitis/tonsillitis, pneumonia

Side effects: Headache, rash, abnormal taste, diarrhea, vomiting, nausea, abdominal pain, dyspepsia, anaphylaxis, anorexia, anxiety

Special considerations:

- The patient should not take this medication with pimozide, cisapride, moxifloxacin, or thioridazine.
- The patient should complete the full course of therapy.
- Biaxin XL should be taken with food.

(152)

Indication: Anxiety disorders

Side effects: Tachycardia, numbness or tingling, tremors, drowsiness, weakness, dry mouth, restlessness, trouble sleeping, headache, nausea, constipation, upset stomach

Special considerations:

- Patients taking this medication should avoid consuming alcohol, grapefruit, or grapefruit juice.
- The patient should wait 14 days before initiating therapy after being on an MAOI or 7 days before taking an MAOI after stopping this medication.

(153)

Brand name: Nizoral

Generic name: Ketoconazole

Drug class: Antifungal, imidazole

- Notice the suffix -*conazole*, which distinguishes antifungals from other drug classes.

(154)

Brand name: VESIcare

Generic name: Solifenacin succinate

Drug class: Bladder antispasmodic

- Relaxes the muscles of the bladder and urinary tract.

(155)

Indications: Tinea corporis, tinea cruris, tinea pedis, tinea versicolor, yeast infections and other fungal infections caused by susceptible organisms

Side effects: Change in hair texture, blisters on scalp, dry skin, oily or dry hair or scalp, irritation, itching, or stinging

Special considerations:

- The oral form of this medication should be taken with food.

- Antacids, proton pump inhibitors and H_2 blockers should be avoided for 2 hours before and after medication administration.

- Topical form of this medication is flammable. It should not be used near an open flame or while smoking.

(154)

Indication: Overactive bladder

Side effects: Dry mouth, constipation, drowsiness, upset stomach, blurred vision, dry eyes, headache, tiredness, weakness

Special considerations:

- This medication may cause drowsiness. Patients should not operate heavy machinery until they know how this medication will affect them.

- Patients should limit consumption of alcohol.

(155)

Brand name: Dolophine

Generic name: Methadone hydrochloride

Drug class: Opiate analgesic, synthetic opioid, N-methyl-D-aspartate (NMDA) receptor antagonist

- Blocks the NMDA receptor.

(156)

Brand name: Minocin

Generic name: Minocycline

Drug class: Semisynthetic tetracycline antibiotic

- Inhibit protein synthesis of susceptible bacteria.

(157)

Indication: Severe chronic pain, addiction to narcotics (such as heroin)

Side effects: Shallow breathing, hallucinations, confusion, chest pain, dizziness, fainting, tachycardia, trouble breathing, lightheadedness, fainting, feeling anxious, restlessness, sleep problems

Special considerations:

- This is a Schedule II habit-forming drug.
- The patient should wait 14 days before initiating therapy after being on an MAOI or 7 days before taking an MAOI after stopping this medication.

(156)

Indication: Treatment of infections caused by susceptible gram-positive and gram-negative organisms

Side effects: Diarrhea, dizziness, drowsiness, indigestion, lightheadedness, loss of appetite, nausea, vomiting

Special considerations:

- Medications that end in the suffix *–cycline* are tetracycline derivative antibiotics.
- Tetracycline can cause permanent discoloration (blue-grey staining) in children under 8 years of age.

(157)

Brand name: Pyridium

Generic name: Phenazopyridine

Drug class: Urinary tract analgesic

- Treats pain associated with the lower urinary tract.

(158)

Brand name: Levitra

Generic name: Vardenafil

Drug class: Phosphodiesterase-5 enzyme (PDE) inhibitor

- Increases blood flow.

(159)

Indication: Relief of symptoms associated with conditions leading to urinary tract irritation

Side effects: Headache, dizziness, stomach pain, skin itching

Special considerations:

- This medication will cause urine to change to an orange-red color.

- This medication should not be used for more than 2 days unless otherwise recommended by a physician.

(158)

Indications: Erectile dysfunction, impotence

Side effects: Flushing, headache, upset stomach, diarrhea, flulike symptoms, nausea, chest pain, hypotension, blurred vision, abnormal ejaculation, priapism

Special considerations:

- This medication may cause drowsiness. Patients should not operate heavy machinery until they know how this medication will affect them.

- Patients should limit consumption of alcohol.

- This medication should not be taken concurrently with nitrates.

(159)

Brand name: Clovate

Generic name: Clobetasol propionate

Drug class: Corticosteroid

- Exhibits anti-inflammatory effects.

(160)

Brand name: Tessalon Perles

Generic name: Benzonatate

Drug class: Non-narcotic antitussive

- Reduces the cough reflex.

(161)

Indication: Various skin conditions including eczema, dermatitis, and psoriasis

Side effects: Itching, burning, irritation, stinging, dryness, redness

Special considerations:

- The usual course of treatment is 7–14 days.

- This medication is not suitable for children under 18 years of age unless otherwise advised by a physician.

(160)

Indication: Relief of nonproductive cough

Side effects: Sedation, headache, mental confusion, visual hallucinations, pruritus, skin eruptions, constipation, nausea, vomiting, stomach upset, nasal congestion, eye irritation, feeling cold, chest numbness

Special consideration:

- This medication should not be given to children under 10 years of age.

(161)

Brand name: Avodart

Generic name: Dutasteride

Drug class: 5-alpha-reductase inhibitor, antiandrogen

- Lowers levels of dihydrotestosterone (DHT) leading to a decrease in the size of the prostate.

(162)

Brand name: Uloric

Generic name: Febuxostat

Drug class: Antigout, xanthine oxidase inhibitor

- Reduces levels of uric acid.

(163)

Indication: Benign prostatic hyperplasia (BPH)

Side effects: Decreased libido, headache, dizziness, drowsiness, nausea, vomiting, constipation, mild itching, skin rash

Special consideration:

- This medication is teratogenic and should not be handled by women who are or may be pregnant.

(162)

Indication: Gout

Side effects: Nausea, joint pain, liver problems, swelling, stiffness, skin rash, dizziness

Special consideration:

- This medication should not be taken concurrently with azathioprine or mercaptopurine.

(163)

Brand names: Pamelor, Aventyl

Generic name: Nortriptyline

Drug class: Tricyclic antidepressant (TCA)

- Treats depression.

(164)

Brand name: Daliresp

Generic name: Roflumilast

Drug class: Phosphodiesterase-4 (PDE-4) inhibitor, anti-inflammatory

- Decreases swelling in the lungs.

(165)

Indications: Depression, anxiety, and tension

Side effects: Nausea, vomiting, loss of appetite, anxiety, insomnia, dry mouth, unusual taste, little or no urination, vision changes, breast swelling, decreased libido, impotence

Special considerations:

- The patient should wait 14 days before initiating therapy after being on a monoamine oxidase inhibitor (MAOI).

- This medication is not approved for use in children.

- This medication should not be stopped abruptly without physician recommendation.

(164)

Indication: Severe chronic obstructive pulmonary disease (COPD)

Side effects: Diarrhea, nausea, dizziness, headache, back pain, muscle spasm, decreased appetite, uncontrollable shaking, insomnia, abdominal pain, rhinitis, sinusitis, urinary tract infection

Special consideration:

- This medication should not be taken concurrently with rifampicin, phenobarbital, carbamazepine, or phenytoin.

(165)

Brand name: AcipHex

Generic name: Rabeprazole

Drug class: Proton pump inhibitor (PPI)

- Prevents acid buildup.

- Notice the suffix *-prazole*, which distinguishes PPIs from other drug classes.

(166)

Brand name: Enbrel

Generic name: Etanercept

Drug class: Antirheumatic, disease-modifying tumor necrosis factor (TNF) blocker

- Decreases levels of a protein produced by the immune system.

(167)

Indications: Gastroesophageal reflux disease (GERD), ulcers, Zollinger-Ellison syndrome

Side effects: Blistering, rash, hives, swelling, difficulty breathing, irregular heartbeat, excessive tiredness, dizziness, lightheadedness, muscle spasms, uncontrollable shaking, seizures, severe diarrhea, stomach pain, fever

Special considerations:

- The patient should not take this medication if hypersensitive to other proton pump inhibitors.

- This medication should be taken 30–60 minutes prior to a significant meal.

- PPIs increase the risk of fracturing wrists, hips, or spine.

- Serious side effects should be reported to the physician.

(166)

Indications: Moderate to severe rheumatoid arthritis, psoriasis, ankylosing spondylitis

Side effects: Headache, erythema, itching, pain, swelling, upper respiratory tract infection, rhinitis, infection, dizziness, rash, abdominal pain, dyspepsia, nausea, vomiting, weakness, sinusitis, cough

Special consideration:

- Patients on Enbrel should avoid receiving live vaccines.

(167)

Brand name: Bystolic

Generic name: Nebivolol

Drug class: Beta blocker, beta$_1$ receptor selective blocker

- Relaxes blood vessels and slows heart rate.

- Notice the suffix -*olol*, which distinguishes beta blockers from other drug classes.

(168)

Brand name: Relafen

Generic name: Nabumetone

Drug class: NSAID

- Nonsteroidal anti-inflammatory drugs (NSAIDs) have antipyretic (fever-reducing), anti-inflammatory, and analgesic (pain relieving) effects.

(169)

Indication: Hypertension

Side effects: Headache, dizziness, tiredness, nausea, slow heartbeat, trouble sleeping

Special considerations:

- Patients should be told to stand up slowly to lessen the chance of orthostatic hypotension.

- Patients should avoid tobacco use and dress warm while on this medication.

(168)

Indications: Pain, swelling, joint stiffness associated with arthritis, gout attacks

Side effects: Upset stomach, nausea, vomiting, constipation, diarrhea, gas, dizziness, drowsiness, headache

Special considerations:

- This medication should not be taken with other medications that also cause bleeding.

- Prolonged use of NSAIDs may increase risk of serious cardiovascular thrombotic events, myocardial infarction, and stroke.

- This medication should be taken with food.

- Patients should be aware that overuse of NSAIDs can lead to serious GI adverse events including bleeding, ulceration, and perforation of the stomach or intestines.

(169)

Brand name: Macrobid

Generic name: Nitrofurantoin

Drug class: Antibiotic

- Treats urinary tract infections (UTIs).

(170)

Brand name: NitroStat SL

Generic name: Nitroglycerin

Drug class: Antianginal, nitrate

- Prevents or relieves chest pain.

(171)

Indication: Bladder infections caused by susceptible bacterial organisms

Side effects: Nausea, headache, vomiting, abdominal pain, yellowing eyes/skin, tiredness, tachycardia, vision changes, new signs of infection, easy bruising, numbness, muscle weakness, lung problems, persistent diarrhea, yeast infection

Special considerations:

- This medication should be taken with food.

- Patients should complete all medication as prescribed by the physician.

- Patients should avoid antacids containing magnesium trisilicate while on this medication.

- This medication may cause urine discoloration (dark yellow to brown). Dark brown urine may have other underlying causes.

- Any persistent or serious side effects should be immediately reported to the physician.

(170)

Indication: Angina

Side effects: Headache, dizziness, lightheadedness, nausea, flushing, burning/tingling under tongue

Special consideration:

- This medication may cause drowsiness. Patients should not operate heavy machinery until they know how this medication will affect them.

(171)

Brand name: Ditropan

Generic name: Oxybutynin

Drug class: Antispasmodic

- Relaxes muscles of the bladder.

(172)

Brand name: Cialis

Generic name: Tadalafil

Drug class: Phosphodiesterase-5 enzyme (PDE) inhibitor

- Relaxes blood vessels in the lungs, thereby increasing blood flow.

(173)

Indication: Overactive bladder

Side effects: Dry mouth, dizziness, drowsiness, blurred vision, dry eyes, nausea, vomiting, upset stomach, abdominal pain, constipation, diarrhea, headache, unusual taste in mouth, dry skin, weakness

Special consideration:

- This medication may cause drowsiness. Patients should not operate heavy machinery until they know how this medication will affect them.

(172)

Indications: Erectile dysfunction, pulmonary arterial hypertension

Side effects: Flushing, diarrhea, myalgia, headache, dyspepsia, insomnia, dizziness, erythema, rash, gastritis, urinary tract infection, abnormal vision, nasal congestion, rhinitis, sinusitis

Special considerations:

- This medication should not be taken concurrently with grapefruit juice.
- This medication should not be used concurrently with nitrates of any form.

(173)

Brand name: Kenalog

Generic name: Triamcinolone

Drug class: Corticosteroid

- Reduces inflammation.

(174)

Brand name: Exelon

Generic name: Rivastigmine

Drug class: Acetylcholinesterase inhibitor, parasympathomimetic, cholinergic

- Stops acetylcholinesterase from destroying the neurotransmitter acetylcholine.

(175)

Indications: Allergic reactions, eczema, psoriasis

Side effects: Skin redness, burning, itching, skin thinning, blistering, stretch marks

Special considerations:

- This medication should be used in sparing amounts.
- Patients should avoid application around eyes.

(174)

Indications: Dementia in Alzheimer's and Parkinson's patients

Side effects: Nausea, vomiting, loss of appetite, heartburn, indigestion, stomach pain, weight loss, diarrhea, constipation, gas, weakness, dizziness, headache, fatigue, tremor, increased sweating, difficulty falling asleep, confusion

Special considerations:

- Capsules should be taken in the evening.
- Patch application sites should be rotated.

(175)

Brand name: Ceftin

Generic name: Cefuroxime

Drug class: Cephalosporin antibiotic (2nd generation)

- Stops the growth of bacteria.

(176)

Brand name: Robaxin

Generic name: Methocarbamol

Drug class: Muscle relaxant

- Helps relax muscles.

(177)

Indication: Infections caused by susceptible bacterial organisms

Side effects: Upset stomach, vomiting, diarrhea, stomach pain, severe skin rash, itching, hives, difficulty breathing, wheezing, diaper rash, painful sores in mouth or throat, vaginal itching and discharge

Special considerations:

- Medication should be completed as prescribed.

- This medication is contraindicated in pregnancy and in patients allergic to penicillin or other cephalosporin agents.

- Antibiotics may decrease effects of oral contraceptives.

(176)

Indications: Muscle spasms, muscle pain

Side effects: Dizziness, drowsiness, headache, confusion, loss of coordination, nausea, vomiting, upset stomach, flushing, blurred vision, insomnia, stuffy nose, rash

Special considerations:

- This medication may cause drowsiness or blurred vision. Patients should not operate heavy machinery until they know how this medication will affect them.

- Patients on this medication should avoid alcohol consumption.

(177)

Brand name: Travatan

Generic name: Travoprost

Drug class: Antiglaucoma agent

- Increases the amount of fluid drainage from the eye.

(178)

Brand name: Latuda

Generic name: Lurasidone

Drug class: Atypical antipsychotic

- Exhibits antagonistic effects on dopamine and serotonin receptors.

(179)

Indications: Open-angle glaucoma and eye hypertension

Side effects: Blurred vision, eye redness, dry eyes, tearing, eyelid crusting, increase in eyelashes, darkening of eyelashes, eyelid changes, photosensitivity

Special consideration:

• This medication may cause blurred vision. Patients should not operate heavy machinery until they know how this medication will affect them.

(178)

Indications: Schizophrenia, depression associated with bipolar disorder

Side effects: Drowsiness, dizziness, nausea, shaking, weight gain, mask-like facial expression, agitation

Special considerations:

• This medication may cause drowsiness. Patients should not operate heavy machinery until they know how this medication will affect them.

• Patients on this medication should avoid alcohol consumption.

(179)

Brand name: Hytrin

Generic name: Terazosin

Drug class: Alpha adrenergic blocker

- Reduces blood pressure by relaxing veins and arteries.
- Promotes easier urination by relaxing muscles of the prostate and the bladder.

(180)

Brand name: Evista

Generic name: Raloxifene

Drug class: Selective estrogen receptor modulator (SERM)

- Treats and prevents osteoporosis by decreasing bone thinning and breakdown.

(181)

Indications: Hypertension, benign prostatic hyperplasia

Side effects: Mild dizziness, weakness, drowsiness, blurred vision, nausea, headache, edema, palpitation, chest pain, dry mouth, dyspnea, nasal congestion

Special considerations:

- This medication may cause drowsiness. Patients should not operate heavy machinery until they know how this medication will affect them.

- Patients on this medication should avoid alcohol consumption.

(180)

Indication: Postmenopause osteoporosis

Side effects: Hot flashes, leg cramps, thromboembolism, edema, arthralgia, leg cramps, muscle spasm, flu syndrome, infection, chest pain, syncope, varicose vein, headache, depression, insomnia, vertigo, fever, migraine, rash, breast pain, nausea, vomiting, weight gain, abdominal pain, diarrhea, dyspepsia, myalgia, arthritis, bronchitis, rhinitis, pharyngitis, pneumonia

Special considerations:

- This medication should not be used by premenopausal women.

- This medication may harm an unborn fetus and should not be handled by women who are, or may become, pregnant. The dust from the tablets should also not be breathed by women who are, or may become, pregnant.

(181)

Brand name: Remeron

Generic name: Mirtazapine

Drug class: Antidepressant, alpha$_2$ adrenergic blocker

- Increases release of norepinephrine and serotonin.

(182)

Brand name: Humira

Generic name: Adalimumab

Drug class: Antirheumatic, disease-modifying, monoclonal antibody, tumor necrosis factor (TNF) blocker

- Acts on TNF receptors, thereby reducing pathologic pain and joint destruction.

(183)

Indication: Depressive illness

Side effects: Somnolence, cholesterol increase, constipation, dry mouth, increase in appetite, weight gain, hypertension, vasodilation, edema, dizziness, abnormal dreams, abnormal thoughts, confusion, vomiting, anorexia, abdominal pain, urinary frequency, myalgia, back pain, arthralgia, tremor, weakness, dyspnea, flulike syndrome, thirst

Special consideration:

- Patients should avoid consumption of alcohol.

(182)

Indications: Rheumatoid arthritis, psoriatic arthritis, ankylosing spondylitis, Crohn's disease, plaque psoriasis

Side effects: Headache, rash, upper respiratory tract infection, sinusitis, hypertension, hyperlipidemia, hypercholesterolemia, nausea, abdominal pain, urinary tract infection, back pain, hematuria, accidental injury, flulike syndrome

Special considerations:

- This medication should not be given to patients with an active chronic infection.
- This medication should not be used concurrently with echinacea.

(183)

Brand name: Cogentin

Generic name: Benztropine

Drug class: Anti-Parkinson's, anticholinergic

- Decreases the effects of acetylcholine and thereby decreases tremors.

(184)

Brand names: Gablofen, Lioresal

Generic name: Baclofen

Drug class: Skeletal muscle relaxant, antispastic

- Relieves muscle spasticity.

(185)

Indications: Parkinson's disease, drug-induced extrapyramidal symptoms (excluding tardive dyskinesia)

Side effects: Tachycardia, confusion, disorientation, memory impairment, toxic psychosis, visual hallucinations, rash, heat stroke, hyperthermia, constipation, dry throat, ileus, nasal dryness, nausea, vomiting, dry mouth, urinary retention, blurred vision, fever

Special considerations:

- Patients on this medication should avoid consumption of alcohol.

- Patients may take this medication with food to decrease gastrointestinal effects.

(184)

Indication: Spasticity caused by multiple sclerosis or spinal cord lesions

Side effects: Drowsiness, vertigo, dizziness, psychiatric disturbances, insomnia, slurred speech, ataxia, hypotonia, weakness, hypotension, fatigue, confusion, headache, rash, nausea, constipation, polyuria

Special consideration:

- Patients taking this medication should avoid consumption of alcohol.

(185)

Brand name: Apresoline

Generic name: Hydralazine

Drug class: Vasodilator

- Relaxes blood vessels, thereby lowering blood pressure.

(186)

Brand name: Bactroban

Generic name: Mupirocin

Drug class: Topical antibiotic, anti-infective

- Stops growth of bacteria.

(187)

Indication: Hypertension

Side effects: Tachycardia, angina pectoris, dizziness, paradoxical hypertension, peripheral edema, flushing, nausea, vomiting, diarrhea, constipation, impotence, conjunctivitis, nasal congestion, dyspnea

Special considerations:

- Patients taking this medication should avoid consumption of alcohol.

- This medication is contraindicated in patients on monoamine oxidase inhibitors (MAOIs).

(186)

Indications: Impetigo and other skin infections caused by susceptible organisms

Side effects: Blistering, itching, redness, peeling, dryness, skin irritation

Special considerations:

- Patients should avoid getting this medication around eyes, nose, mouth, or damaged skin unless recommended by a physician.

- Patients should follow up with the physician if the condition does not improve in 3–5 days.

(187)

Brand names: Inderal, Inderal LA, InnoPran XL

Generic name: Propranolol

Drug class: Antiarrhythmic, beta adrenergic blocker (nonselective)

- Blocks the action of epinephrine and norepinephrine on beta receptors located mainly in the heart and kidneys.

- Notice the suffix *-olol*, which distinguishes beta blockers from other drug classes.

(188)

Brand name: Chantix

Generic name: Varenicline

Drug class: Nicotinic receptor partial agonist

- Blocks nicotine's effects in the brain.

(189)

Indications: Hypertension, angina pectoris, tremors, arrhythmia, tachycardias, prevention of cardiac arrest, prevention of migraine headache, cardiomyopathy

Side effects: Nausea, vomiting, diarrhea, constipation, stomach cramps, decreased sex drive, impotence, insomnia, fatigue

Special considerations:

- Patients should avoid consumption of alcohol because it may increase propranolol levels in the blood.

- This medication should not be discontinued abruptly.

(188)

Indication: Smoking cessation

Side effects: Nausea, headache, vomiting, drowsiness, gas, constipation, trouble sleeping, unusual dreams, changes in taste

Special considerations:

- This medication should be taken with a full glass of water after eating food.

- Patients on this medication should limit alcohol consumption.

- This medication may cause drowsiness. Patients should not operate heavy machinery until they know how this medication will affect them.

(189)

Brand names: Lotrimin, Cruex, Gyne-Lotrimin, Mycelex, Desenex, Femcare, FungiCURE, Fungoid, Gynix, Pedesil, Trivagizole

Generic name: Clotrimazole

Drug class: Antifungal

- Kills fungal cells by acting on the fungal cell wall and altering the permeability.

(190)

Brand names: Dilantin, Phenytek, Dilantin-125, Cerebyx

Generic name: Phenytoin

Drug class: Anticonvulsant, antiepileptic

- Treats and prevents seizures.

(191)

Indication: Infections caused by susceptible fungal organisms

Side effects: Itching, burning, irritation, redness, swelling, stomach pain, fever

Special consideration:

- This medication should be fully completed unless otherwise advised by a physician.

(190)

Indications: Trigeminal neuralgia, epilepsy, peripheral neuropathy, subarachnoid hemorrhage, encephalitis

Side effects: Insomnia, uncontrollable eye movements, abnormal body movements, loss of coordination, confusion, slowed thinking, slurred speech, dizziness, headache, nausea, vomiting, constipation, unwanted hair growth, enlargement of lips, gingival hyperplasia, penile pain

Special considerations:

- This medication may cause drowsiness. Patients should not operate heavy machinery.
- Patients should maintain good oral hygiene to reduce risk for gingival hyperplasia.
- Patients on this medication should avoid alcohol consumption.

(191)

Brand name: Mirapex

Generic name: Pramipexole dihydrochloride

Drug class: anti-Parkinson, dopamine agonist

- Acts on dopamine receptors and is used to treat the symptoms of Parkinson's disease.

(192)

Brand name: Victoza

Generic name: Liraglutide

Drug class: Antidiabetic (r-DNA injection)

- Lowers blood sugar levels.

(193)

Indications: Parkinson's disease, restless legs syndrome

Side effects: Somnolence, dyskinesia, hallucinations, insomnia, dizziness, nausea, constipation

Special considerations:

- Patients who develop sudden daytime "sleep attacks" should discontinue this medication.

- This medication should be gradually discontinued.

- Extended-release tablets should not be chewed, crushed, or divided.

(192)

Indication: Non-insulin dependent diabetes (Type 2 diabetes)

Side effects: Headache, nausea, diarrhea, bladder pain, bloody or cloudy urine, cough or hoarseness, painful urination, fever or chills, feeling of discomfort, joint pain, loss of appetite, lower back or side pain, muscle aches, runny nose, shivering, sore throat, sweating, insomnia, fatigue, vomiting

Special considerations:

- This medication may increase the risk of developing a thyroid tumor.

- This medication should be stored in the refrigerator.

(193)

Brand name: Brilinta

Generic name: Ticagrelor

Drug class: Antiplatelet

- Inhibits activation and aggregation of platelets.

(194)

Brand name: Onglyza

Generic name: Saxagliptin

Drug class: Antihyperglycemic, hypoglycemic, antidiabetic, dipeptidyl peptidase-4 inhibitor (DPP-4 inhibitor)

- Lowers blood glucose levels by stimulating the release of insulin and decreasing glucagon secretion.
- Improves glycemic control in adjunct to diet and exercise.

(195)

Indication: Acute coronary syndrome

Side effects: Bleeding, dyspnea, headache, dizziness, nausea

Special considerations:

- This medication may cause dizziness. Patients should not operate heavy machinery until they know how this medication will affect them.

- Alcohol may increase the risk for stomach bleeding. Patients should limit consumption of alcohol.

(194)

Indication: Type 2 diabetes mellitus (non-insulin-dependent diabetes)

Side effects: Sore throat, headache, urinary tract infection, gastroenteritis, joint pain, rash, hives, skin peeling, swelling, difficult breathing, hoarseness, vomiting, loss of appetite

Special consideration:

- Notice the suffix *-gliptin*, which distinguishes DPP-4 inhibitors from other drug classes.

(195)

Brand name: Juxtapid

Generic name: Lomitapide

Drug class: Synthetic lipid-lowering agent, cholesterol-lowering agent

- Reduces blood levels of "bad" cholesterol.

(196)

Brand name: Zanaflex

Generic name: Tizanidine

Drug class: Skeletal muscle relaxant

- Relaxes muscles, thereby decreasing spasms and increasing muscle tone.

(197)

Indication: Homozygous familial hypercholesterolemia

Side effects: Vomiting, gas, indigestion, stomach pain, diarrhea, constipation, chest pain, weight loss

Special considerations:

- Patients should avoid grapefruit and grapefruit juice while on this medication.

(196)

Indications: Spasms caused by multiple sclerosis, stroke, brain, or spinal injury

Side effects: Dizziness, drowsiness, weakness, nervousness, depression, vomiting, tingling sensation, dry mouth, constipation, diarrhea, stomach pain, heartburn, muscle spasms, back pain, rash, sweating

Special considerations:

- This medication may cause drowsiness. Patients should not operate heavy machinery until they know how this medication will affect them.

- Patients on this medication should avoid alcohol consumption.

(197)

Brand name: Adderall XR

Generic name: Amphetamine/dextroamphetamine XR

Drug class: Central nervous system stimulant

- Excites the nervous system.

(198)

Brand name: Zostavax

Generic name: Zoster vaccine

Drug class: Vaccine

- Composed of a weakened chickenpox virus (varicella-zoster virus).

(199)

Indications: Narcolepsy, attention deficit hyperactivity disorder (ADHD)

Side effects: Dizziness, hypertension, insomnia, confusion, nausea, diarrhea

Special considerations:

- This is a Schedule II habit-forming drug.
- The patient should not take concurrently with monoamine oxidase inhibitors (MAOIs).
- Patients with hypertension and advanced arteriosclerosis should avoid this medication.

(198)

Indication: Prevention of herpes zoster (shingles) in individuals who are 50 years of age or older

Side effects: Redness, pain, itching, swelling, hard lump, warmth, bruising at site of injection, headache, allergic reactions, chickenpox, fever, hives at the injection site, joint pain, muscle pain, nausea, rash, shingles, swollen glands near injection site

Special consideration:

- This vaccine is contraindicated in children.

(199)

Brand name: Vytorin

Generic name: Ezetimibe/simvastatin

Drug class: Antihyperlipidemic, HMG CoA reductase inhibitor and cholesterol absorption inhibitor

- Lowers high cholesterol and triglyceride levels while increasing good cholesterol levels.

(200)

Indication: High cholesterol

Side effects: Headache, diarrhea, cold symptoms, bloating, chills, constipation, darkened urine, fast heartbeat, fever, hives, hoarseness, indigestion, itching, joint pain, loss of appetite, nausea, abdominal pain, redness of skin, dyspnea, stiffness, swelling, vomiting

Special considerations:

- This medication may harm an unborn fetus or cause birth defects.

- Patients should avoid eating or drinking grapefruit while on this medication.

(200)

absorption

(201)

aerosol

(202)

Absorption is the process of drug entry into the bloodstream.

(201)

An aerosol is a type of dispensing system that contains pressurized active ingredients that are dispersed as mist, spray, or foam upon activation of the product.

(202)

angiotensin-converting enzyme (ACE) inhibitor

(203)

An ACE inhibitor is a classification of drugs that block angiotensin I from being converted to angiotensin II by the angiotensin-converting enzyme. This, in turn, reduces blood pressure and improves heart function. Angiotensin II can cause vasoconstriction that leads to high blood pressure.

Indications: Controls high blood pressure, treats heart failure, prevents strokes, prevents kidney damage, improves survival after heart attacks

Side effects: Cough, hyperkalemia, low blood pressure, dizziness, headache, drowsiness, weakness

Popular ACE inhibitors:

- benazePRIL (Lotensin)
- captoPRIL (Capoten)
- enalaPRIL (Vasotec)
- fosinoPRIL (Monopril)
- lisinoPRIL (Prinivil, Zestril)
- quinaPRIL (Accupril)
- ramiPRIL (Altace)

Notes:

- Note the suffix *-pril*, which distinguishes ACE inhibitors from other drug classes.
- ACE inhibitors interact with lithium and NSAIDs.

(203)

agonist

(204)

An agonist is a chemical agent that interacts with a cell receptor and stimulates a certain action or response.

(204)

alpha-adrenergic blocker

(205)

An alpha-adrenergic blocker, or alpha antagonist, is a classification of drugs that block the alpha receptors. This results in relaxation of smooth muscle and an increase in blood flow and therefore lower blood pressure.

Alpha receptors are found on vascular and nonvascular smooth muscle in both the central and peripheral nervous system. Alpha$_1$ receptors are mostly found postsynaptically in the central nervous system and serve an excitatory function. However, they serve an inhibitory function peripherally. Alpha$_2$ receptors only have inhibitory functions and are found both pre- and postsynaptically. Alpha receptors are activated by epinephrine, norepinephrine, or dopamine.

Indications: Cardiac arrhythmias, hypertension, anxiety, panic disorders

Side effects: Postural hypotension, tachycardia, sedation, nasal stuffiness, miosis

Popular alpha blockers:

- doxazOSIN (Cardura)
- prazOSIN (Minipress)
- tamsulOSIN (Flomax)
- terazOSIN (Hytrin)

Notes:

- Note the suffix -*osin*, which distinguishes alpha blockers from other drug classes.
- These drugs should not be used with other antihypertensives or vasodilators.

(205)

aminoglycoside

(206)

An aminoglycoside is a classification of antibiotic drugs that have bactericidal effects on most gram-negative bacteria. They are usually given intravenously (IV).

Indication: Severe infections due to gram-negative bacteria

Side effects: Dizziness, loss of appetite, increased thirst, muscle twitching, nausea, vomiting, renal toxicity, ototoxicity

Popular aminoglycosides:

- amikaCIN (Amikin)
- gentaMICIN (Garamycin)
- kanaMYCIN (Kantrex)
- paromoMYCIN (Paromycin)
- streptoMYCIN (Ambistryn-S)
- tobraMYCIN (Nebcin)

Note:

- Aminoglycosides generally end with the suffixes *-micin* or *-mycin*. Do not confuse them with macrolide antibiotics, which end with the suffix *-romycin*.

(206)

angiotensin II receptor antagonist or blocker (ARB)

(207)

antagonist

(208)

An ARB is a classification of drugs that help relax blood vessels and thereby lower blood pressure by preventing angiotensin II from attaching to the angiotensin II receptors. Angiotensin II is a chemical that stimulates vasoconstriction and increases blood pressure.

Indications: High blood pressure, diabetic nephropathy, congestive heart failure

Side effects: Cough, hyperkalemia, hypotension, vertigo, headache, drowsiness, diarrhea, rash

Popular angiotensin II receptor blockers:

- candeSARTAN (Atacand)
- irbeSARTAN (Avapro)
- loSARTAN (Cozaar)
- olmeSARTAN (Benicar)
- telmiSARTAN (Micardis)
- valSARTAN (Diovan)

Note:

- ARBs generally end with the suffix -*sartan*, which distinguishes them from other drug classes.

(207)

An antagonist, also known as a blocker, is a chemical agent that attaches to receptors and results in blocking effects. Antagonists do not have any biological effects on a receptor; instead, they just occupy a space, preventing other chemicals from attaching to the blocked receptor.

(208)

antidiabetic

(209)

An antidiabetic is a therapeutic classification of drugs used in the treatment of diabetes to lower blood glucose levels. These medications can be injectable or oral. Insulin injectable is used in the treatment of non-insulin-dependent diabetes mellitus (NIDDM), or type 1 diabetes, which occurs early in childhood and cannot be prevented. Insulin-dependent diabetes mellitus (IDDM), or type 2 diabetes, is most common in adults that are suffering from obesity. Oral medications are used in the treatment of type 2 diabetes; insulin therapy is recommended only for severe cases. This type of diabetes can be prevented with exercise and lifestyle changes. Type 2 antidiabetics include sulfonylureas, alpha-glucosidase inhibitors, biguanides, meglitinides, and thiazolidinediones.

Indication: Diabetes

Side effects: Hypoglycemia, hyperglycemia, nausea, vomiting, gastrointestinal upset

Popular antidiabetics:

- acarbose (Precose)
- GLImepiride (Amaryl)
- GLIpizide (Glucotrol)
- GLYburide (DiaBeta, Micronase)
- insulin R (Humilin R)—rapid acting, type 1 diabetes
- insulin lispro (Humalog)—rapid acting, type 1 diabetes
- isophane insulin suspension (Humulin N)—intermediate acting, type 1 diabetes
- insulin glargine (Lantus)—long acting, type 1 diabetes
- metformin (Glucophage)
- pioGLItazone (Actos)
- repaGLInide (Prandin)

Notes:

- Antidiabetics generally have *gli* or *gly* as a prefix or a word root.
- Glucagon is the antidote for hypoglycemia.
- Not more than 1 mL of insulin can be added to an IV bag.

(209)

antiemetic

(210)

An antiemetic is a therapeutic classification of drugs that treat or prevent nausea and vomiting.

Indications: Emesis, vertigo, emesis prophylaxis

Side effects: Restlessness, drowsiness, fatigue, dry mouth, blurred vision, nausea, diarrhea, sedation

Popular antiemetics:

- chlorpromAZINE (Thorazine)
- dimenhydrinate (Dramamine)
- diphenhydrAMINE (Benadryl)
- dolaSETRON (Anzemet)
- dronabinol (Marinol)—Schedule III controlled substance used mainly in cancer patients
- graniSETRON (Kytril)
- mecliZINE (Antivert)
- metocloprAMIDE (Reglan)
- ondanSETRON (Zofran)
- prochlorperAZINE (Compazine)
- promethAZINE (Phenergan)
- transdermal scopolAMINE (Transderm-Scop)
- trimethobenzAMIDE (Tigan)

Note:

- Antiemetics end with the suffixes *-zine*, *-amine*, *-setron*, or *-amide.*

(210)

antiepileptic (AEDs) or anticonvulsant

(211)

Antiepileptic is a therapeutic classification of medications that suppress neurons from firing rapidly, thereby stopping seizures. These include benzodiazepines, barbiturates, succinimides, and hydantoins.

Indications: Epileptic seizures, neuropathic pain, bipolar disorder

Side effects: Blurred vision, drowsiness, dizziness, nausea, sleepiness

Popular anticonvulsants:

- carbamaZEPINE (Tegretol)
- gabapentin (Neurontin)
- lamotrigine (Lamictal)
- oxcarbaZEPINE (Trileptal)
- phenyTOIN (Dilantin)—hydantoin
- primidone (Mysoline)
- valproic acid (Depakene)
- zonisamide (Zonegran)

Notes:

- Hydantoins end in the suffix *-toin*. Other miscellaneous anticonvulsants have the suffix *-zepine*.
- Patients should be aware that nonprescription drugs should not be used concurrently unless authorized by the physician.

(211)

antihistamine, H_1 antagonist, or H_1 blocker

(212)

An antihistamine is a therapeutic classification of drugs that counteract the effects of histamine, which is released in response to allergic reactions and produces an inflammatory response. Antihistamines exert anticholinergic effects on the body.

Indications: Allergic rhinitis, seasonal allergies, allergic conjunctivitis, allergic reactions to drugs, sedation

Side effects: Dry mouth, drowsiness, dizziness, nausea and vomiting, restlessness or moodiness (in some children), lack of urination, blurred vision, confusion

Popular antihistamines:

- azelastINE (Astelin, Astepro nasal sprays), azelastINE (Optivar eyedrops)
- certirizINE (Zyrtec)
- desloratadINE (Clarinex)
- diphenhydramINE (Benadryl)
- fexofenadINE (Allegra)
- hydroxyzINE (Atarax, Vistaril)
- loratadINE (Claritin, Alavert)
- promethazINE (Anergan, Phenergan)

Notes:

- Most antihistamines end with the suffix *-ine*.
- First-generation antihistamines have a sedative effect but Benadryl may elicit hyperactive behavior in children.

(212)

antihyperlipidemic or antilipemic

(213)

An antihyperlipidemic is a therapeutic classification of drugs that reduce the level of low-density lipoproteins (LDL) cholesterol in the blood. These include: bile acid sequestrants, HMG-CoA (3-hydroxy-3-methyl-glutaryl-CoA) reductase inhibitors or statins, and fibric acid derivatives.

Indications: Hyperlipidemia, atherosclerosis

Side effects: Nausea, vomiting, constipation, abdominal pain or cramps, headache, rhabdomyolysis in toxic conditions

Popular antihyperlipidemic:

- atorvaSTATIN (Lipitor)—HMG-CoA reductase inhibitor
- cholestyramine (Questran)—bile acid sequestrant
- colesevelam HCl (Welchol)—bile acid sequestrant
- fenoFIBRate (Tricor)—fibric acid derivative
- gemFIBRozil (Lopid)—fibric acid derivative
- lovaSTATIN (Mevacor)—HMG-CoA reductase inhibitor
- pravaSTATIN (Pravachol)—HMG-CoA reductase inhibitor
- simvaSTATIN (Zocor)—HMG-CoA reductase inhibitor

Notes:

- HMG-CoA reductase inhibitors end in the suffix *-statin* and are also known as *statins*. Fibric acid derivatives are distinguished from other drug classes by the word root *fibr-*.
- Statins can interact with antacids and antifungals.

(213)

antineoplastic or anticancer

(214)

An antineoplastic is a therapeutic classification of drugs used in the treatment of cancer. The term *chemotherapy* is usually used in reference to treatment with antineoplastic drugs. These include alkylating agents, antibiotics, antimetabolites, antimitotic agents, biologic modifiers, hormones, monoclonal antibodies, platinum complexes, and topoisomerase inhibitors.

Indications: Various types of cancer

Side effects: Bone marrow suppression, diarrhea, fatigue, headaches, nausea, vomiting, loss of hair (alopecia)

Popular antineoplastics:

- carboPLATIN (Paraplatin)—platinum complex
- cisPLATIN (Platinol-AQ)—platinum complex
- cycloPHOSPHAMIDE (Cytoxan)—alkylating agent
- doceTAXEL (Taxotere)—mitotic inhibitor
- doxoruBICIN (Adriamycin, Doxil)—antibiotic
- erloTINIB (Tarceva)—epidermal growth factor receptor (EGFR) inhibitor
- eTOPOSIDE (Toposar)—topoisomerase inhibitor
- 5-FluoroURACIL or 5-FU (Adrucil)—antimetabolite
- gemCITABINE (Gemzar)—antimetabolite
- hydroxyUREA (Droxia, Hydrea)—antimetabolite
- irinOTECAN (Camptosar)—topoisomerase inhibitor
- methoTREXATE (Trexall, Rheumatrex)—antimetabolite
- pacliTAXEL (Taxol)—mitotic inhibitor
- topOTECAN (Hycamtin)—topoisomerase inhibitor
- vinBLASTINE (Velban)—mitotic inhibitor
- vinCRISTINE (Oncovin, Vincasar)—mitotic inhibitor

Notes:

- Monoclonal antibodies generally end in the suffix -*mab*. Examples include bevacizuMAB and rituxiMAB.
- Other antineoplastics have the suffixes -*platin, -phosphamide, -taxel, -bicin, -tinib, -uracil, -citabine, -toposide, -otecan, -trexate, -blastine,* or -*cristine.*

(214)

antipyretic

(215)

Antipyretic agents exhibit fever relieving effect. The most common antipyretics are acetaminophen and nonsteroidal anti-inflammatory drugs (NSAIDs). NSAIDs have antipyretic, anti-inflammatory, and analgesic (pain-relieving) effects.

Indication: Fever

Side effects: Stomach upset, nausea, heartburn, ulcers of the stomach, gastritis

Popular antipyretics:

- acetaminoPHEN (Tylenol)
- acetyl salicylic acid (Aspirin)
- ibuproFEN (Motrin)
- naproxen (Aleve)

Note:

- Antipyretics are some of the most commonly used drugs on the market and should be easy to remember.

(215)

antitussive

(216)

Antitussives are medications that exhibit cough-suppressant effects.

Indication: Dry or nonproductive coughs caused by colds, flu, or lung infections

Side effects: Slowed or difficulty breathing, severe drowsiness, rash or itching, upset stomach, constipation, nervousness or restlessness

Popular antitussives:

- benzonatate (Tessalon Perles)
- bromPHENiramine, dextromethorPHAN, guaiFENesin, and pseudoEPHEDRINE (AccuHist DM)
- chlorPHENiramine, dextromethorPHAN, and pseudoEPHEDRINE (Creomulsion cough)
- chlorPHENiramine, dihydrocodeine, and PHENylephrine (Novahistine DH liquid)—Schedule III
- dextromethorPHAN (Benylin, Delsym, Hold DM, Percussion CS children)
- dextromethorPHAN and guaiFENesin (T-Tussin DM)
- guaiFENesin and codeine (Robitussin ac)—Schedule V

Notes:

- Most antitussives have *-phen*, *-fen*, *-phan*, or *ephedrine* as part of their names.
- Antitussives should not be used concurrently with MAOIs. There should be a minimum of 2 weeks between ending an MAOI therapy and initiating antitussives.
- Over-the-counter cold and cough medicine should not be given to children younger than 4 years of age due to serious side effects.

(216)

aseptic technique/USP 797

(217)

Aseptic technique means *without or absence of the presence of microorganisms*. United States Pharmacopoeia (USP) chapter 797 gives enforceable guidelines for the preparation of sterile products or compounded sterile products (CSPs) in an effort to prevent contamination. It emphasizes the importance of compounding in a cleanroom with a positive pressure environment, training of personnel, and quality assurance. Hazardous substances are to be compounded in a cleanroom with a negative pressure environment. USP 797 also sets guidelines for beyond-use dating of CSPs that align with the compounding environment and sterility.

The risk of contaminating USPs is divided into three risk levels as follows:

Low risk or risk level 1: Preparing simple admixtures in a sterile environment which require minimal manipulation (Example: Advantage bags, mini-bag plus).

Medium risk or risk level 2: Preparing batch products in a sterile environment using complex manipulations or multiple additives. This includes the preparation of parenteral nutrition solutions using automated devices.

High risk or risk level 3: Preparation of products using nonsterile ingredients or nonsterile final containers (nuclear pharmaceuticals). This includes reconstitution of products in an environment with air quality less than ISO Class 5.

Cleanrooms and laminar flow hoods are classified using the International Organization for Standardization (ISO) classes, which are based on the number of particles bigger than half a micron present in a cubic foot of air. The six classes are:

- Class 1 (ISO 3)—A class 1 cleanroom or ISO 3 would not contain more than 1 particle bigger than half a micron in every cubic foot of air.
- Class 10 (ISO 4)
- Class 100 (ISO 5)
- Class 1000 (ISO 6)
- Class 10000 (ISO 7)
- Class 100000 (ISO 8)

(217)

bacteriocidal

(218)

bacteriostatic

(219)

A bacteriocidal is an agent that has "cidal" effects, or that can kill bacteria.

(218)

Bacteriostatic medications are agents that inhibit the growth of bacteria by stopping them from reproducing.

(219)

barbiturate

(220)

A barbiturate is a classification of drugs that once used to be the first-line treatment for anxiety and insomnia. Today, benzodiazepines are preferable because they are safer to use.

Indications: Mild sedation, general anesthesia, seizure disorders

Side effects: Anxiety, nausea, drowsiness, lack of coordination, respiratory depression, potential for abuse

Popular barbiturates:

- mephoBARBITAL (Mebaral)—Schedule IV
- phenoBARBITAL (Luminal)—Schedule IV
- pentoBARBITAL (Nembutal)—Schedule II
- secoBARBITAL (Seconal)—Schedule II

Notes:

- Barbiturates have the suffix -*barbital*.
- These drugs interact with antipsychotic medications, corticosteroids, oral contraceptives, blood-thinning medications, the antibiotic doxycycline, and anticonvulsants.

(220)

benzodiazepine

(221)

A benzodiazepine is a classification of drugs that have sedative and hypnotic properties.

Indications: Sedation, insomnia, anxiety, muscle spasticity, involuntary movement disorders, convulsions

Side effects: Increased anxiety, drowsiness, hostility, irritability, confusion, skin rash, nausea, headache, lack of coordination, vertigo, potential for abuse

Popular benzodiazepines:

- alpraZOLAM (Xanax)—Schedule IV
- chlordiazepoxide (Librium)—Schedule IV
- clonaZEPAM (Klonopin)—Schedule IV
- diaZEPAM (Valium)—Schedule IV
- loraZEPAM (Ativan)—Schedule IV
- midaZOLAM (Versed)—Schedule IV
- oxaZEPAM (Serax)—Schedule IV
- temaZEPAM (Restoril)—Schedule IV

Notes:

- Most benzodiazepines end with the suffix *-zepam, or -zolam.*
- All benzodiazepines belong to the DEA schedule IV.
- These drugs should not be taken with alcohol because they cause drowsiness.

(221)

beta-adrenergic blocking agent or beta blocker

(222)

A beta blocker is a classification of drugs that block the beta receptors. There are three beta receptors known as: $beta_1$, $beta_2$, and $beta_3$. $Beta_1$ receptors are mainly found in the heart and in the kidneys. $Beta_2$ receptors are mainly in the lungs, gastrointestinal tract, vascular smooth muscle, and skeletal muscle. However, the $beta_3$ receptors are only located in fat tissue. Beta blockers can be $beta_1$ or $beta_2$ selective and would act exclusively on either of the receptors or they can be nonselective and act on both $beta_1$ and $beta_2$ receptors.

Indications: Abnormal heart rhythm, high blood pressure, heart failure, angina, tremor

Side effects: Hypotension, dizziness, headache, tiredness, depression, diarrhea, pruritus, bradycardia, dyspnea, cold extremities, constipation, dyspepsia, heart failure, hypotension, nausea, wheezing

Popular beta blockers:

- atenOLOL (Tenormin)—$beta_1$ selective blocker
- carvediLOL (Coreg)—nonselective agent
- labetaLOL (Normodyne, Trandate)—nonselective agent
- metoprOLOL (Lopressor)—$beta_1$ selective blocker
- propranOLOL (Inderal)—nonselective agent
- sotaLOL (Betapace)—nonselective agent

Notes:

- Beta blockers generally end with the suffix *-olol*.
- These medications should not be discontinued abruptly without the recommendation of a physician.

(222)

bioavailability

(223)

bioequivalent

(224)

black box warning/adverse drug event

(225)

Bioavailability is a term that refers to the level of availability of a certain drug at the site of action or the target tissue.

(223)

Bioequivalent is a term that refers to the equivalence of the active ingredients of a generic drug to the respective brand name. In pharmacy, the orange book is used as a reference for therapeutic equivalence of generic drugs.

(224)

Adverse drug events are side effects that are unwanted and undesirable effects of a drug on the body. The desirable effects would be called *therapeutic effects*.

The FDA can require a pharmaceutical company to place a black box warning on the package insert of medications that may cause serious or possibly life-threatening side effects to warn the consumer of the health risks.

Usually, the black box warning would be composed of text inside a black box frame and placed at the top of the package insert.

(225)

bronchodilator

(226)

A bronchodilator is a classification of drugs that dilate or expand the bronchi and bronchioles, allowing more air to flow into the lungs. These medications include beta$_2$ agonists, anticholinergics, and xanthine derivatives.

Indications: Bronchial asthma, chronic bronchitis, emphysema

Side effects: Restlessness, anxiety, hypertension, palpitations, cardiac arrhythmias, insomnia

Popular bronchodilators:

- albuTEROL (Proventil HFA, Ventolin HFA)—sympathomimetic
- aminoPHYLLINE (Phyllocontin)—xanthine derivative
- ipraTROPIUM (Atrovent)—anticholinergic
- ipraTROPIUM and albuTEROL (Combivent)—sympathomimetic
- levalbuTEROL (Xopenex)—sympathomimetic
- salmeTEROL (Serevent)—sympathomimetic
- terbuTALINE (Brethine)—sympathomimetic
- theoPHYLLINE (Theo-dur)—xanthine derivative

Notes:

- Bronchodilators have the suffixes *-terol*, *-tropium*, *-taline*, or *-phylline.*
- Other bronchodilators used for asthma include corticosteroids and leukotriene-receptor antagonists, which are oral medications and include monteLUKAST (Singulair) and zafirLUKAST (Accolate).

(226)

cephalosporin

(227)

A cephalosporin is a classification of antibiotics that interfere with the bacterial cell wall and are usually bacteriocidal.

Indication: Infections caused by susceptible bacteria

Side effects: Pruritus, urticaria, skin rashes, dizziness, heartburn, fever, cough, muscular aches and pains, headache, hepatic and renal dysfunction, aplastic anemia (decrease in red blood cell production), epidermal necrolysis

Popular cephalosporins:

- CEFazolin (Ancef, Kefzol)—first generation
- CEFaclor (Ceclor)—second generation
- CEFotetan (Cefotan)—second generation
- CEFoxitin (Mefoxin)—second generation
- CEFuroxime (Ceftin)—second generation
- CEFdinir (Omnicef)—third generation
- CEFepime (Maxipime)—third generation
- CEFtazidime (Frotaz)—third generation
- CEFtriaxone (Rocephin)—third generation
- CEPHalexin (Keflex)—first generation

Notes:

- Cephalosporins generally have the prefix *cef-* or *ceph-*.
- They should not be used in patients that are allergic to penicillins.

(227)

contraindication

(228)

A contraindication is a condition that renders a medication undesirable.

(228)

corticosteroid

(229)

A corticosteroid is a classification of anti-inflammatory drugs that include steroid hormones naturally synthesized by the adrenal cortex and their synthetic analogs.

Indications: Asthma, chronic bronchitis, rheumatoid arthritis, inflammatory bowel disease

Side effects: Mood swings, glaucoma, hyperglycemia, hypertension, fluid retention, weight gain

Popular corticosteroids:

- betamethasONE (Celestone)
- cortisONE (Cortone)
- dexamethasONE (Decadron)
- fludrocortisONE (Florinef)
- hydrocortisONE (Cortef)
- methylprednisOLONE (Solu-Medrol, Medrol)
- prednisOLONE (Pediapred, Orapred)
- prednisONE (Deltasone)

Notes:

- Most corticosteroids end with the suffix *-one* or *-olone*. They also may have the root *cort*.
- These drugs are not indicated for long-term use.

(229)

diluent

(230)

A diluent is a solvent, usually water, added to a solution to reconstitute it or to reduce its concentration; the smaller the concentration of a solution, the larger the volume and vice versa.

(230)

diuretic

(231)

A diuretic is a classification of drugs that increase the secretion of water by the kidneys. These include carbonic anhydrase inhibitors, loop diuretics, osmotic diuretics, potassium-sparing diuretics, and thiazides.

Indications: Edema associated with congestive heart failure, kidney and liver diseases, hypertension

Side effects: Hypokalemia, diarrhea, nausea, vomiting, drowsiness, electrolyte imbalance, dehydration, hypotension, uric acid retention, hyperkalemia associated with the potassium-sparing diuretics, ototoxicity associated with loop diuretics

Popular diuretics:

- acetaZOLAMIDE (Diamox)—carbonic anhydrase inhibitor used in treatment of glaucoma
- bumeTANIDE (Bumex)—loop diuretic
- furoSEMIDE (Lasix)—loop diuretic
- hydrochloroTHIAZIDE (HydroDiuril)—thiazide diuretic
- isoSORBIDE (Ismotic)—osmotic diuretic
- mannitol (Osmitrol)—osmotic diuretic
- metOLAZONE (Zaroxolyn)—thiazide diuretic
- spironoLACTONE (Aldactone)—potassium-sparing diuretic
- torSEMIDE (Demadex)—loop diuretic

Notes:

- Most diuretics end with the suffixes *-zolamide*, *-tanide*, *-semide*, *-sorbide*, *-lactone*, or *-olazone*.
- These medications should not be stopped unless advised by a physician.
- Patients should avoid alcohol while taking these drugs.

(231)

elixir

(232)

emulsion

(233)

enteral

(234)

An elixir contains active ingredients combined with a sweetened and flavored alcoholic or hydroalcoholic base intended for oral use.

(232)

An emulsion is a mixture formed of liquids that are immiscible using an emulsifying agent.

(233)

The enteral route of drug administration requires medications to be absorbed through the gastrointestinal system before being distributed throughout the body. Rectal route (PR), sublingual (SL), and the oral routes are enteral. The following are parenteral routes:

Inhalation	(INH)
Intradermal	(ID)
Intramuscular	(IM)
Intravenous	(IV)
Intrathecal	(IT)
Subcutaneous	(SC, SQ)

(234)

expectorant

(235)

fluoroquinolone or quinolone

(236)

An expectorant or a mucolytic is a medication that thins the mucus so it may be easier to expel the mucus from the chest. This is usually recommended for dry or nonproductive cough. Expectorants include the following medications:

- guaifenesin liquid (Robitussin)
- guaifenesin tablet (Mucinex)

(235)

A fluoroquinolone is a group of broad-spectrum antibiotics, which means that they are effective against both gram-negative and gram-positive bacteria.

Indication: Treatment of infection caused by susceptible bacteria

Side effects: Nausea, diarrhea, headache, abdominal pain or discomfort, dizziness

Popular fluoroquinolones:

- ciproflOXACIN (Cipro)
- gatiflOXACIN (Tequin)
- levoflOXACIN (Levaquin)
- moxiflOXACIN (Avelox)

Notes:

- Fluoroquinolones generally end with the suffix -*oxacin*.
- Ciprofloxacin is effective against anthrax infection.
- Fluoroquinolones should not be used concurrently with anticoagulants, antacids, and NSAIDs.

(236)

histamine H$_2$ antagonist

(237)

H_2 antagonists block the release of histamine at the H_2 receptors located in the stomach. This in turn reduces the secretion of gastric acid and relieves heartburn.

Indications: Gastric or duodenal ulcers, gastric hypersecretion disorders, gastroesophageal reflux disease (GERD)

Side effects: Dizziness, somnolence, headache, confusion, hallucinations, diarrhea

Popular H_2 antagonists:

- cimeTIDINE (Tagamet)
- famoTIDINE (Pepcid)
- nizaTIDINE (Axid)
- raniTIDINE (Zantac)

Notes:

- H_2 antagonists end with the suffix *-tidine*.
- There are many drug–drug interactions with the H_2 antagonist medications. These include interactions with antacids, anticoagulants, antimetabolites, and alkylating agents.

(237)

indication

(238)

macrolide

(239)

An indication is a medical use of a drug. For example, acetaminophen is indicated for headaches.

(238)

A macrolide is a classification of broad-spectrum drugs that can be bacteriostatic or bacteriocidal in susceptible organisms.

Indications: Bacterial infections due to susceptible organisms, respiratory tract infections, in patients with penicillin allergy

Side effects: Nausea, vomiting, diarrhea, abdominal pain

Popular macrolides:

- azithROMYCIN (Zithromax)
- clarithROMYCIN (Biaxin)
- dirithROMYCIN (Dynabac)
- erythROMYCIN (E-mycin, Eryc)

Notes:

- Notice the suffix -*romycin*, which distinguishes macrolide antibiotics from other drug classes.
- These medications should be taken with food.

(239)

monoamine oxidase inhibitor (MAOI)

(240)

An MAOI is a classification of drugs that exhibit antidepressant effects by inhibiting the actions of the monoamine oxidase enzyme responsible for the breakdown of norepinephrine, serotonin, and dopamine at the synapse.

Indications: Used in patients with atypical depression who do not respond well or are allergic to other antidepressants

Side effects: Drowsiness, postural hypotension, arrhythmias, dry mouth, constipation, urinary retention

Popular MAOIs:

- phenelzINE (Nardil)
- selegilINE (Eldepryl)
- tranylcypromINE (Parnate)

Notes:

- Most MAOIs end with the suffix -*ine*.
- MAOIs interact with a lot of other drugs and also foods containing tyramine (certain cheeses, meats, alcoholic beverages, fruits, and vegetables).
- MAOIs should not be taken concurrently with TCAs or SSRIs.
- There should be a period of 14 days between stopping MAOIs and initiating alternative therapy using other antidepressants.

(240)

parenteral

(241)

The parenteral route of drug administration bypasses the gastrointestinal system so drugs enter the bloodstream directly. The parenteral route is efficient in emergency situations but allows little time to reverse the effects of drugs in case of overdose or allergic reactions.

Parenteral routes include the following:

- Inhalation
- Intradermal (ID)
- Intramuscular (IM)
- Intravenous (IV)
- Subcutaneous (SC)
- Sublingual (SL)
- Topical
- Transdermal

(241)

proton pump inhibitor (PPI)

(242)

A proton pump inhibitor is a classification of drugs that block the last step of acid production, thereby suppressing acid secretion.

Indications: Treatment of *Helicobacter pylori* (H. pylori), gastric disorders, gastric and duodenal ulcers, GERD, gastric acid hypersecretory conditions

Side effects: Headache, diarrhea, abdominal pain, nausea, flatulence, constipation, dry mouth

Popular proton pump inhibitors:

- esomePRAZOLE (Nexium)
- lansoPRAZOLE (Prevacid)
- omePRAZOLE (Prilosec)
- pantoPRAZOLE (Protonix)
- rabePRAZOLE (Aciphex)

Notes:

- PPIs end with the suffix *-prazole*.
- PPIs are generally taken in the morning on an empty stomach, which increases their absorption.

(242)

psychomotor stimulant

(243)

A psychomotor stimulant is a classification of central nervous system (CNS) stimulant drugs that, among other effects, increase heart rate and blood pressure and disrupt sleep. These include amphetamines and nonamphetamine behavioral stimulants.

Indications: Narcolepsy, attention deficit hyperactivity disorder (ADHD)

Side effects: High blood pressure, arrhythmias, restlessness, tremor, anxiety, irritability, headache, dizziness, insomnia, dry mouth

Popular psychomotor stimulants:

- AMPHETAMINE, dextroAMPHETAMINE mixed salts (Adderall)—Schedule II
- dextroAMPHETAMINE (Dexedrine)—Schedule II
- methylPHENidate (Ritalin)—Schedule II
- moDAFINIL (Provigil)—Schedule IV
- pemoline (Cylert)—Schedule IV
- siBUTRAMINE (Meridia)—Schedule IV

Notes:

- Most psychomotor stimulants have the suffix *-amphetamine, -butramine,* or *-dafinil* and they may have the word root *phen-*.
- All psychomotor stimulants are scheduled drugs and have potential for abuse.
- Psychomotor stimulants interact with antihypertensives, tricyclic antidepressants, and foods high in tyramine content.

(243)

selective serotonin reuptake inhibitor (SSRI)

(244)

An SSRI is a classification of drugs that inhibit the reuptake of serotonin at the synapse. They are used as first-line treatment for depression.

Indications: Major depression, obsessive–compulsive disorders (OCD), anxiety

Side effects: Anxiety, headache, nervousness, dizziness, insomnia, nausea, vomiting, weight loss, sweating, rash, pharyngitis

Popular SSRIs:

- citalOPRAM (Celexa)
- dulOXETINE (Cymbalta)
- escitalOPRAM (Lexapro)
- fluOXETINE (Prozac)
- fluvOXAMINE (Luvox)
- parOXETINE (Paxil)
- sertraLINE (Zoloft)

Notes:

- SSRIs generally end with the suffixes *-opram, -oxetine,* or *-oxamine.*
- SSRIs should not be taken at the same time as MAOIs or TCAs due to serious, life-threatening side effects.

(244)

solvent

(245)

sulfonamide or sulfa drug

(246)

A solvent is an inactive medium, usually water, used to dissolve solutes or solid particles (active ingredients). In semisolids, the inactive medium or base can be petroleum jelly or Eucerin.

(245)

A sulfonamide is a classification of bacteriostatic antibiotics that were discovered in 1935 by German Gerhard Domagk before the discovery of penicillins.

Indications: Urinary tract infections (UTIs), inflammation of the middle ear, ulcerative colitis, lower respiratory tract infections

Side effects: Hematologic disorders, anorexia, urticaria (hives), pruritus (itching), photosensitivity, nausea, vomiting, diarrhea, abdominal pain, chills, fever

Popular sulfonamides:

- SULFAdiazine (Silvadene)
- SULFAmethoxazole and trimethoprim (Bactrim, Septra)
- SULFAsalazine (Azulfidine)
- SULFisoxazole (Gantrisin)

Notes:

- Sulfonamides generally have the prefix *sulfa-*.
- These medications should be taken with plenty of water and on an empty stomach 1–2 hours before a meal.
- Patients should be advised to avoid sunlight while on these medications.

(246)

syrup

(247)

tetracycline

(248)

A syrup consists of active ingredients mixed with a base of concentrated solution of sugar in water.

(247)

A tetracycline is a group of bacteriostatic antibiotics that are chemically composed of a four-ring structure. Hence, they are named *tetra*cyclines.

Indications: Acne, Rickettsiae fever, chronic bronchitis, Lyme disease

Side effects: Nausea, vomiting, diarrhea, epigastric distress, skin rashes, photosensitivity

Popular tetracyclines:

- doxyCYCLINE (Vibramycin)
- minoCYCLINE (Monodox)
- tetraCYCLINE (Achromycin, Sumycin)

Notes:

- Tetracyclines generally end with the suffix *-cycline*.
- They should not be used in children younger than 9 years of age because they may lead to permanent discoloration of teeth.
- Tetracyclines used beyond their expiration date would exhibit toxic effects.

(248)

tincture

(249)

tricyclic antidepressant (TCA)

(250)

A tincture is an alcoholic or hydroalcoholic solution containing pure chemical substances or plant extractions.

(249)

A TCA is a classification of drugs used in the treatment of depression. However, they are not indicated as first-line treatment. TCAs are chemically composed of a three-ringed structure and hence the name *tri*cyclic.

Indications: Depression, concurrently with analgesics in neuropathic pain

Side effects: Sedation, dry mouth, orthostatic hypotension, mental confusion, lethargy, disorientation, rash, nausea, vomiting, urinary retention, constipation, photosensitivity

Popular TCAs:

- amiTRIPTYLINE (Elavil)
- clomiPRAMINE (Anafranil)
- desiPRAMINE (Norpramin)
- doXEPIN (Sinequan)
- imiPRAMINE (Tofranil)
- norTRIPTYLINE (Pamelor)

Notes:

- TCAs generally end with the suffixes *-triptyline,* or *-pramine.*
- These medications should not be used in children younger than 12 years of age, with the exception of imipramine, which was found to be helpful in children with bedwetting problems.

(250)

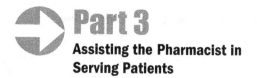

Part 3

Assisting the Pharmacist in Serving Patients

What is the body surface area for a child who is 90 lb and 165 cm tall?

A. 1.3 m²
B. 1.4 m²
C. 4.7 m²
D. 2.2 m²

(251)

B. 1.4 m²

Rationale:

$$BSA~(m^2) = \sqrt{\frac{([\,Height~(cm)\times Weight~(kg)\,])}{3,600}} ~~or~ \sqrt{\frac{([\,Height~(in)\times Weight~(lb)\,])}{3,131}}$$

Method 1: Convert weight into kilogram using proportions: 1 kg = 2.2 lb

So $\dfrac{1~kg}{2.2~lb} = \dfrac{x}{90~lb}$ and solve for x:

$$x = \frac{(1~kg \times 90~lb)}{2.2~lb} = 40.9~kg$$

Then, plug the numbers into the appropriate equation:

$$\sqrt{\frac{([\,40.9~(cm)\times 165(kg)\,])}{3,600}} = \sqrt{\frac{([6748.5])}{3,600}} = \sqrt{1.87} = 1.4~m^2$$

Method 2: Convert height into inches: 1 in. = 2.54 cm,

so $\dfrac{1~in.}{2.54~cm} = \dfrac{x}{165~cm}$ and solve for x:

$$x = \frac{(165~cm \times 1~in.)}{(2.54~cm)} = 64.96~in.$$

Then, plug the numbers into the appropriate equation:

$$\sqrt{\frac{([\,64.96~(in)\times 90~(lb)\,])}{3,131}} = \sqrt{\frac{([5846.5])}{3,131}} = \sqrt{(1.87)} = 1.4~m^2$$

(251)

A medication that has an expiration date of 12/14 would expire on:

A. the last day of December 2014
B. 12/01/14
C. 12/14/14
D. December of 2012

(252)

In the NDC 4253-4221-11, what is represented by the second set of numbers?

A. the manufacturer
B. the package size
C. the product name, strength, and dosage form
D. the number of tablets in the medication package

(253)

A. the last day of December 2014

Rationale:

Medications expire at midnight on the last day of the expiration month designated by the manufacturer unless the exact expiration date is specified on the medication label. So, if a medication has an expiration of 12/14, it will expire on 12/31/14 at midnight.

(252)

C. the product name, strength, and dosage form

Rationale:

The NDC number is 10 digits long and comprised of three sets of numbers that are divided as follows:

1. The first set can be comprised of 4 to 5 digits and represents the manufacturer.

2. The second set is comprised of 3 to 4 digits and represents the product name, strength, and dosage form.

3. The third set is comprised of 2 digits and represents the package size.

(253)

The *Orange Book* is most often used to find:

A. compatibility of medications given parenterally
B. average wholesale prices
C. manufacturer's standards
D. therapeutic equivalents

(254)

A pharmacy technician's scope of practice includes all of the following EXCEPT:

A. refilling medications
B. answering patients' questions regarding their medications
C. answering insurance-related questions
D. reviewing prescription orders for accuracy of information

(255)

D. therapeutic equivalents

Rationale:

- The *Injectable Drug Handbook* is a reference source for compatibility of medications given parenterally.

- The *Red Book* is a reference source for the average wholesale prices.

- The manufacturer's standards are referenced in the *Physician's Desk Reference (PDR)*, which is a compilation of package inserts for FDA-approved drugs.

- The *Orange Book* is a reference source for therapeutic equivalents.

(254)

B. answering patients' questions regarding their medications

Rationale:

Only pharmacists can counsel patients regarding their medications.

(255)

Which of these drugs does not belong to the penicillin class
of antibiotics?

A. Unasyn
B. Augmentin
C. tetracycline
D. PenVee K

(256)

A pharmacy technician is given 120 mL of a 20% dextrose
solution and is told to dilute it with 6 oz of sterile water.
What would be the final percent concentration?

A. 13%
B. 8%
C. 14%
D. 20%

(257)

C. tetracycline

Rationale:

Unasyn (ampicillin/sulbactam), Augmentin (amoxicillin clavulanate), and PenVee K (penicillin V-potassium or PenVee K) all belong to the penicillin class of antibiotics. Tetracycline belongs to the tetracycline class of antibiotics.

(256)

B. 8%

Rationale:

1 oz = 30 mL, so 6 oz = 6 × 30 mL = 180 mL

Use the dilution equation:

Concentration 1 (C1) × Quantity (Q1) = Concentration (C2) × Quantity (Q2)

C1 = 20%, Q1 = 120 mL, Q2 = 180 mL + 120 mL = 300 mL

20% (120 mL) = x (300 mL)

x = 2,400/300 = 8%

(257)

Which act distinguished between legend and nonlegend drugs?

A. the 1951 Durham Humphrey Amendment
B. the 1962 Kefauver-Harris Amendment
C. the 1983 Orphan Drug Act
D. the 1914 Harrison Narcotic Act

(258)

What is the maximum number of refills permitted for a Schedule III medication?

A. no refills are allowed
B. six refills within 5 months, whichever occurs first
C. five refills within 6 months, whichever occurs first
D. three refills within 90 days

(259)

A. the Durham Humphrey Amendment

Rationale:

- The Durham Humphrey Amendment distinguished between prescription and over-the-counter (nonlegend) drugs prohibiting the sale of legend (prescription) drugs without a prescription.

- The Kefauver-Harris Amendment requires drugs to be proven pure, safe, and effective.

- The Orphan Drug Act encourages finding drug treatments for rare (orphaned) diseases.

- The Harrison Narcotic Act limits the transport, manufacture, and sale of opium and any of its derivatives. It requires a written prescription to purchase any of the aforementioned drugs.

(258)

C. five refills within 6 months, whichever occurs first

Rationale:

Schedule III–V medications can be refilled up to five times within 6 months, whichever occurs first. Thereafter, a new prescription is required.

(259)

A pharmacy technician receives a prescription that reads 2 gtt AU BID. What will the label placed on the patient's medication read?

A. two drops in both ears two times daily
B. two drops in both eyes two times daily
C. two drops in the right ear three times a day
D. two drops in the left eye two times daily

(260)

A. two drops in both ears two times daily

Rationale:

2 gtt: 2 drops

AU: Both ears

BID: Twice a day

Be careful not to confuse AU with OU, which means both eyes. Here are some other abbreviations to watch out for:

OD: Right eye (Latin: oculus dexter)

OS: Left eye (Latin: oculus sinister)

AD: Right ear (Latin: aurio dexter)

AS: Left ear (Latin: aurio sinister)

Remember that "O" is for ophthalmic and "A" is for ear.

(260)

What is CCXLIX equivalent to?

A. 254
B. 269
C. 240
D. 249

(261)

D. 249

Rationale:

C = 100

C = 100 = same value as the letter to its immediate left

The addition rule applies:

C + C = 100 + 100 = 200

X = 10

L = 50 = larger value than the letter to its immediate left

The subtraction rule applies:

L − X = 50 − 10 = 40

I = 1

X = 10 = larger value than the letter to its immediate left

The subtraction rule applies:

X − I = 10 − 1 = 9

Then add all the values: 200 + 40 + 9 = 249.

(261)

Glyburide is classified into which drug class?

A. anticonvulsant
B. hypertension
C. antidiabetic
D. proton pump inhibitor

(262)

Reducing a substance to fine particles using a mortar and pestle is known as which of the following?

A. blending
B. triturating
C. sifting
D. tumbling

(263)

C. antidiabetic

Rationale:

Glyburide (Diabeta) is an oral antidiabetic.

(262)

B. triturating

Rationale:

- Blending is the mixing together of two different substances until a homogenous mixture is achieved.

- Triturating is the breaking down of compounds into finer particles.

- Sifting is the process of eliminating large particles by using a sifter.

- Tumbling is the process of mixing by adding different ingredients into a bag or a jar and shaking them until a homogenous mixture is achieved.

(263)

Which of the following is an automated dispensing machine?

A. Omnicell
B. Baker Cell
C. Kirby Lester
D. both A and B

(264)

How many days will the following prescription last?

Famotidine 20 mg #120

Sig: Famotidine 40 mg po BID

A. 28 days
B. 30 days
C. 32 days
D. 34 days

(265)

A. Omnicell

Rationale:

Accu-Dose, Omnicell, Pyxis, and ScriptPro are all automated dispensing machines. Baker Cell and Kirby Lester are digital pill-counting machines.

(264)

B. 30 days

Rationale:

Famotidine 40 mg BID is equivalent to 4 tablets per day. Since the quantity dispensed is 120, divide that number by the number of tablets the patient will be receiving per day (4) to find out how many days the prescription will last. In summary:

(total number of tablets) ÷ (number of tablets to be taken per day) = number of days the tablets will last: (120) ÷ (4) = 30 days

(265)

How old must a person be to purchase an exempt narcotic?

A. 12 years
B. 16 years
C. 18 years
D. 21 years

(266)

Which of the following statements regarding sterile compounding is true?

A. A barrier isolator or a horizontal laminar flow hood can be used to compound IV antibiotics.
B. Compounded sterile products (CSPs) are also known as extemporaneous compounding.
C. A horizontal laminar flow hood can be used for compounding chemotherapy.
D. A laminar flow hood is cleaned using bleach and water.

(267)

C. 18 years

Rationale:

Individuals purchasing exempt narcotics or Schedule V narcotics have to be 18 years of age or older. The quantity of purchase, the date of purchase, and the residential address of the purchaser are recorded by the dispensing pharmacist. Mailing addresses such as P. O. box numbers are not acceptable because they can be changed often.

(266)

A. A barrier isolator or a horizontal laminar flow hood can be used to compound IV antibiotics.

Rationale:

- A barrier isolator or glove box and the horizontal laminar flow hood can be used to compound IV antibiotics.

- Extemporaneous compounding are non-commercially available and nonsterile products that are prepared for specific patient needs in response to a physician's prescription. These include ointments, creams, liquids, and so on.

- Hazardous products such as chemotherapy can only be compounded under a vertical flow hood or a barrier isolator with negative pressure.

A laminar flow hood is cleaned with sterile water followed by 70% isopropyl alcohol.

(267)

Which of the following statements is true regarding measurement of liquid using a graduated cylinder?

A. Liquids are measured at eye level by reading the top of the meniscus.

B. Liquids that form an upside-down meniscus are measured at eye level by reading the lowest point.

C. Liquids that form an upside-down meniscus are measured at eye level by reading the midpoint between the top and the bottom of the meniscus.

D. Liquids are measured at eye level by reading the bottom of the meniscus.

(268)

D. Liquids are measured at eye level by reading the bottom of the meniscus.

Rationale:

To measure liquids in a graduated cylinder, one must read at eye level the lower portion of the meniscus. The meniscus is the concave shape that forms at the top of the graduated cylinder because of liquid's affinity to glass.

If the liquid forms an upside-down or convex meniscus, one must read at eye level the highest point of the meniscus.

(268)

Which of the following regulations gives enforceable guidelines for the preparation of sterile products to prevent contamination?

A. Pure Food and Drug Act of 1906
B. Poison Prevention Packaging Act of 1970
C. USP 797
D. FDA Safe Medical Devices Act of 1990

(269)

Which of the following information is required on the medication label of a prepackaged or repackaged unit-dose medication in an inpatient setting?

A. patient's name, date of birth, name of medication, and direction of use
B. medication name and strength, lot number, and expiration date
C. medication name and strength, lot number, and directions for use
D. patient's name, pharmacy name and address, physician's name, and the number of refills

(270)

C. USP 797

Rationale:

- The Pure Food and Drug Act of 1906 prohibits the sale of misbranded and adulterated foods and drugs.

- The Poison Prevention Packaging Act of 1970 requires all medications to be packaged in childproof containers to prevent accidental child poisoning. However, patients who sign a waiver are exempt from this regulation. Also, certain emergency medications such as nitroglycerin sublingual are dispensed in non-childproof packaging.

- United States Pharmacopoeia (USP) chapter 797 gives enforceable guidelines for the preparation of sterile products or compounded sterile products (CSPs) in an effort to prevent contamination. It emphasizes the importance of compounding in a cleanroom with a positive pressure environment, training of personnel, and quality assurance. USP 797 also sets guidelines for beyond use dating of CSPs that align with the compounding environment and sterility.

- The FDA Medical Devices Act of 1990 requires reporting serious injuries and deaths caused by medical equipment to the FDA and the manufacturer.

(269)

B. medication name and strength, lot number, and expiration date

Rationale:

Unit-dose packages must have the following information: medication name, dosage form and strength, manufacturer's name, the repackaging lot number, and the repackaging expiration date.

(270)

Which of the following is an example of an aminoglycoside?

A. tobramycin
B. amoxicillin
C. penicillin
D. Augmentin

(271)

If the strength of a drug is omitted from the prescription, your duty as a pharmacy technician would be to:

A. tell the pharmacist
B. call the doctor
C. guess what strength the drug is supposed to be, because you know the patient's diagnosis
D. input the strength that is most ordered for this drug

(272)

A. tobramycin

Rationale:

Amoxicillin, penicillin, and Augmentin (amoxicillin and clavulanate) belong to the penicillin class of antibiotics.

(271)

A. tell the pharmacist

Rationale:

When in doubt, consult the pharmacist. Do not attempt to guess on a medication order because that can only lead to medication errors.

(272)

How often can a patient refill a Schedule II prescription?

A. one time
B. twice within 1 year
C. as needed
D. no refills

(273)

What is the flow rate of 1,000 mL of 0.45% sodium chloride solution infused over 12 hours?

A. 7 mL/hr
B. 50 mL/hr
C. 83 mL/hr
D. 125 mL/hr

(274)

D. no refills

Rationale:

Schedule II medications cannot be refilled even if a written prescription indicated an infinite amount of refills. The prescription may be partially filled if the pharmacy is unable to supply the full quantity because of stock shortage, for example. However, the remainder should be supplied to the patient within 72 hours or a new prescription will be needed. The patient will have the choice of receiving the full quantity at a different pharmacy.

(273)

C. 83 mL/hr

Rationale:

Use the following equation:

flow rate = (total volume) ÷ (total hours)

(1,000 mL) ÷ (12 hours) = 83 mL/hr

Always round to a whole number. The infusion rate is never indicated by a decimal number.

(274)

What is required during preparation of chemotherapy?

A. double gloving
B. compounding under a horizontal flow hood
C. compounding on a counter top in an open area
D. using filter needles

(275)

A. double gloving

Rationale:

- Double gloving is the most important part of donning personal protective equipment (PPE) in preparation for mixing chemotherapy.

- Compounding under a horizontal flow hood is reserved to nonhazardous agents. Chemotherapy should be compounded under a vertical flow hood.

- Compounding chemotherapy on a countertop in an open area would lead to airborne emissions of cytotoxic drugs into the local atmosphere.

- Filter needles are used during the preparation of products from ampoules and they are not a requirement for chemotherapy preparation unless medication is withdrawn from ampoules.

(275)

What is 0.45% NS?

A. 0.45% normal strength
B. half normal saline
C. 0.45% nonstop
D. 0.45% nonstandard

(276)

B. half normal saline

Rationale:

- $D_{10}W$ = 10% dextrose in water
- D_5W = 5% dextrose in water
- 0.45% NS = Half normal saline or 0.45% normal saline
- 0.9% NS = Normal saline or 0.9% normal saline
- $D_5\frac{1}{2}NS$ = Dextrose 5% with 0.45% normal saline
- D_5NS = Dextrose 5% with 0.9% normal saline
- $D_5\frac{1}{4}NS$ = Dextrose 5% with a quarter or 0.25% normal saline
- SWFI = Sterile water for irrigation
- LR = Lactated Ringer's solution

(276)

Which of the following is the net cost of medications paid by a pharmacy after applying all adjustments and discounts?

A. capitation fee
B. copay fee
C. actual acquisition cost
D. dispensing fee

(277)

Which method would be the most accurate for determining the appropriate pediatric dose?

A. Young's rule
B. Clark's rule
C. drug-specific information from the manufacturer
D. BSA formula

(278)

C. actual acquisition cost

Rationale:

- A capitation fee is a set amount of money received by a pharmacy from an insurance company per patient regardless of the number of prescriptions filled per year.

- A copay is a fee paid by the patient at the time of purchase.

- The actual acquisition cost (AAC) is the net cost of medications paid by a pharmacy after applying all adjustments and discounts.

- A dispensing fee is the cost of filling a prescription incurred by a pharmacy. This includes employee salaries, overhead, and the overall cost of preparing and dispensing the medication.

(277)

C. drug-specific information from the manufacturer

Rationale:

- Pharmacy technicians should always refer to information from the manufacturer or package insert for the most accurate drug-specific information.

- Young's and Clark's rules are now outdated and hardly ever used.

- The BSA formula is useful in determining the patient's BSA or the appropriate dose based on the BSA if an adult dose is given. However, without the drug-specific information, this would be useless.

(278)

Which of the following is invalid regarding airflow in a horizontal laminar flow hood?

A. The air flows from the back of the hood toward the compounder.
B. The expelled air ejected toward the compounder is picked up by the pre-filter and recycled through the high-efficiency particulate air (HEPA) filter.
C. Hanging an IV bag over a reconstituted vial may lead to obstruction of air flow.
D. Air flow may be obstructed creating a zone of turbulence or backwash when two objects are placed in front of one another inside the laminar flow hood.

(279)

Work area is designated by how many inches from the front edge and the sides of the laminar airflow hood?

A. 6 inches from the front edge and 3 inches from the sides
B. 6 inches from the front edge and 6 inches from the sides
C. 5 inches from the front edge and 5 inches from the sides
D. 8 inches from the front edge and 6 inches from the sides

(280)

C. Hanging an IV bag over a reconstituted vial may lead to obstruction of air flow.

Rationale:

Hanging an IV bag over a reconstituted vial may lead to obstruction of air flow in a vertical air flow hood. The rest of the statements apply to the horizontal laminar flow hood.

In a horizontal laminar air flow hood, the air flows horizontally from the high-efficiency particulate air (HEPA) filter in the back to the front toward the compounder.

In a vertical flow hood, the air flows vertically from the HEPA filter on top to the compounding surface at the bottom.

(279)

B. 6 inches from the front edge and 6 inches from the sides

Rationale:

The designated work surface area inside a laminar airflow hood is 6 inches from the edge and 6 inches from the sides to guard against contamination.

(280)

All of the following vitamins are fat-soluble EXCEPT:

A. vitamin A
B. vitamin B
C. vitamin D
D. vitamin K

(281)

What is the most important thing to remember when preparing products using an ampoule?

A. to use an ampoule breaker
B. to wipe the ampoule with an alcohol swab
C. to use a filter needle to draw up the solution and to change the needle when injecting the solution into the IV bag or vice versa
D. to use a Luer-Lok syringe

(282)

B. vitamin B

Rationale:

Only B and C vitamins are water soluble. Vitamins A, D, E, and K are fat soluble.

(281)

C. to use a filter needle to draw up the solution and to change the needle when injecting the solution into the IV bag or vice versa

Rationale:

It is of utmost importance to remember to use a filter needle or a filter straw when drawing up solution from an ampoule. It is also crucial to change the needle before transferring the solution into an IV bag because the needle used first could be contaminated with glass particles. One can start off by using a regular needle to draw up the solution and then change to a filter needle to transfer the solution into the IV bag. The solution needs to be filtered using a 5 micron filter to eliminate all glass particles.

(282)

How would 8:30 p.m. be expressed in military time?

A. 2130
B. 1830
C. 2030
D. 2050

(283)

Which of the following procedures must be followed to prevent coring?

A. insert the needle into the vial with the bevel tip down
B. insert the needle into the vial with the lumen side up
C. insert the needle at a 45°–60° angle
D. both B and C

(284)

C. 2030

Rationale:

Military time is based on a 24-hour time interval starting with midnight (which is 0000 or 2400) to eliminate the confusion associated with the use of a.m. and p.m. Morning hours are denoted with zeroes in the front. For example: 1:00 a.m. becomes 0100. After 12 noon or 1200, a 100 is added to denote each following hour. For example: 1:00 p.m. becomes 1300 and so on.

(283)

D. both B and C

Rationale:

Coring means that a piece of the vial's rubber stopper broke off and entered the drug. Caution should be exercised to prevent coring. If coring is suspected, the solution should be filtered before transfer into the IV bag. Inserting the needle into the vial with the lumen (opening) side up at a 45°–60° angle can reduce the chances of coring the rubber stopper.

(284)

Which of these statements is true?

A. The larger the needle gauge, the larger the diameter of the needle.
B. The larger the needle gauge, the longer the diameter of the needle.
C. The larger the needle gauge, the smaller the diameter of the needle.
D. The larger the needle gauge, the shorter the diameter of the needle.

(285)

What are the base components of a hyperalimentation admixture?

A. amino acids and dextrose
B. amino acids, dextrose, and proteins
C. amino acids, dextrose, and electrolytes
D. amino acids, dextrose, multivitamins, and trace elements

(286)

C. The larger the needle gauge, the smaller the diameter of the needle.

Rationale:

As the needle gauge increases, the diameter of the needle decreases. So, a 28-gauge (G) needle is smaller than a 16-gauge needle.

(285)

A. amino acids and dextrose

Rationale:

The base of a hyperalimentation or parenteral nutrition admixture is composed of amino acids and dextrose or amino acids, dextrose, and lipids combinations. Amino acids provide the patient with protein and dextrose with energy. Electrolytes, vitamins, minerals, and trace elements are additives and not base components.

(286)

A vertical laminar flow hood is reserved for the preparation of which of the following?

A. antibiotic IV piggybacks
B. hazardous agents
C. antibiotic irrigation solutions
D. creams and ointments

(287)

What is the generic name for Concerta?

A. etomidate
B. valsartan
C. lopressor
D. methylphenidate

(288)

B. hazardous agents

Rationale:

A vertical laminar flow hood is reserved for preparation of hazardous agents such as chemotherapy.

(287)

D. methylphenidate

Rationale:

- Etomidate is the generic name for Amidate.

- Valsartan is generic for Diovan.

- Metoprolol is the generic name for Lopressor.

(288)

Which of the following is an antineoplastic medication?

A. amikacin
B. doxepin
C. doxorubicin
D. erythromycin

(289)

Which of the following is an anticonvulsant medication?

A. etoposide
B. carbamazepine
C. sulfadiazine
D. glipizide

(290)

C. doxorubicin

Rationale:

- Amikacin is an aminoglycoside.
- Doxepin is a tricyclic antidepressant.
- Erythromycin is a macrolide antibiotic.

(289)

B. carbamazepine

Rationale:

- Etoposide is an antineoplastic.
- Sulfadiazine is a sulfa antibiotic.
- Glipizide is an antidiabetic.

(290)

If a drug is ordered 1 cap TID × 20 days; what would be the total quantity needed to complete the medication regimen?

A. 3 capsules
B. 20 capsules
C. 1 capsule
D. 60 capsules

(291)

How much codeine is found in Tylenol #3?

A. 8 mg
B. 15 mg
C. 30 mg
D. 60 mg

(292)

D. 60 capsules

Rationale:

1 cap TID × 20 days = 1 capsule three times a day for 20 days

To find out the number of capsules needed to complete the medication therapy, first find out how many capsules are to be taken per day and then multiply that number by the total number of days:

(1 × 3) = 3 capsules per day

3 capsules per day × 20 days = 60 capsules total over 20 days

(291)

C. 30 mg

Rationale:

- Tylenol #1 contains 8 mg of codeine and 325 mg of acetaminophen.

- Tylenol #2 contains 15 mg of codeine and 300 mg of acetaminophen.

- Tylenol #3 contains 30 mg of codeine and 300 mg of acetaminophen.

- Tylenol #4 contains 60 mg of codeine and 300 mg of acetaminophen.

(292)

What is the generic name for Tenormin?

A. atenolol
B. carvedilol
C. albuterol
D. metoprolol

(293)

An FDA recall of a product that is not likely to result in any adverse health consequences is known as:

A. class I recall
B. class II recall
C. class III recall
D. class IV recall

(294)

A. atenolol

Rationale:

- The generic name for Tenormin is atenolol.

- Carvedilol is the generic name for Coreg.

- Albuterol is the generic name for ProAir, Ventolin, and Proventil.

- Metoprolol is the generic name for Lopressor.

(293)

C. class III recall

Rationale:

- A class I recall indicates that a serious adverse health consequence or death may occur.

- A class II recall indicates that a temporary or reversible adverse health consequence may occur.

- A class III recall indicates that it is not likely that any adverse health consequences will occur.

- There is no such thing as a class IV recall.

Recalls are issued by the FDA or the manufacturer. Recalls should be pulled from stock, returned to the wholesaler or manufacturer, and reordered. To identify the recalled batch, the lot number of the medication is the most useful piece of information.

(294)

A pharmacy technician receives an order for amoxicillin 20 mg per kg every 12 hours. The patient is a child who weighs 40 lb and whose height is 120 cm. The medication is available in a concentration of 400 mg/5 mL. How much amoxicillin will the patient receive per day?

A. 20 mL
B. 9 mL
C. 10 mL
D. 4.5 mL

(295)

B. 9 mL

Rationale:

Step 1: Convert the weight of the patient from pounds to kilograms:

1 lb = 2.2 kg, so 1 kg = 2.2 lb, so 1 kg/2.2 lb = x/40 lb and
x = (1 kg × 40 lb)/2.2 lb = 18.18 kg

Step 2: Calculate the dose in milligrams:

18.18 kg × 20 mg/kg = 363.6 mg per dose

Or 20 mg/2.2 lb = x/40 lb

x = 363.6 mg per dose

Step 3: Calculate amount of medication patient is to receive per day:

363.6 mg every 12 hours = 363.6 mg × 2 = 727.2 mg

Remember there are 24 hours in a day, so every 12 hours would be twice a day.

Step 4: Calculate amount of medication in milliliters:

400 mg/5 mL = 727.2 mg/x

x = 9 mL per day or 4.5 mL per dose

(295)

While filling a medication order, you notice that a patient who is allergic to penicillin is ordered tobramycin 80 mg. Furthermore, the patient's profile shows that gentamicin 60 mg is an active order. You alert the pharmacist because:

A. there is an allergic cross-sensitivity between penicillin and tobramycin
B. there is a drug–drug interaction between tobramycin and gentamicin
C. there is an allergic cross-sensitivity between penicillin and gentamicin
D. all of the above

(296)

B. there is a drug–drug interaction between tobramycin and gentamicin

Rationale:

Tobramycin and gentamicin are both aminoglycosides and should not be administered at the same time because this may lead to serious adverse effects including liver toxicity. The pharmacy technician should alert the pharmacist about the interaction so that the physician is contacted about discontinuing one of the medications. There is no allergic cross-sensitivity between penicillin and gentamicin or penicillin and tobramycin.

(296)

A patient who is taking Lipitor finds out that she is pregnant. Lipitor is FDA pregnancy category X. What should the patient do?

A. continue the course of the medication because there is no evidence of risk to the fetus

B. continue using the medication because the benefits outweigh the potential risks

C. stop taking the medication immediately and tell the physician because this medication may lead to fetal abnormalities

D. none of the above

(297)

C. stop taking the medication immediately and tell the physician because this medication may lead to fetal abnormalities

Rationale:

FDA pregnancy categories are as follows:

- Category A: The patient can continue to take the medication since studies do not show any risk to the fetus.

- Category B: The patient can continue to take the medication but should be aware that there are no adequate human studies, although animal studies do not show any fetal risk.

- Category C: The patient should be aware that she should take this medication only if the benefits outweigh the potential risks.

- Category D: The patient should take the medication only if the benefits outweigh the potential risks in life-threatening situations in which safer drugs cannot be used.

- Category X: The patient should be aware that this medication is contraindicated in pregnancy and should not be taken.

(297)

A geriatric patient who weighs 150 lb is ordered vancomycin (Vancocin) 30 mg/kg/24 hr IV in two equally divided doses. How much medication will the patient receive per dose?

A. 2 g
B. 1 g
C. 1,200 mg
D. 1.2 g

(298)

B. 1 g

Rationale:

Step 1: Convert weight from pounds to kilograms:

1 kg/2.2 lb = x/150 lb

$x = (150 \times 1)/2.2 = 68.18$ kg

Step 2: Find out how much medication the patient will receive per dose.

Since the dose is 30 mg/kg/24 hr in two equally divided doses, one dose is equal to 15 mg/kg/12 hr:

15 mg/kg = x/68.18 kg

$x = 1022.7$ mg per dose = 1.02 g per dose or 1 g per dose

Hint: One can also calculate the amount of medication received by the patient per day by using 30 mg/kg/24 hr and then dividing the answer by 2 to find out how much medication the patient is receiving per dose.

(298)

A cancer patient with hematologic toxicity is ordered leucovorin 20 mg/m² every 6 hours. The patient is 180 lb and 5'10". How much medication will the patient receive per day?

A. 1,636 mg
B. 40 mg
C. 160 mg
D. 240 mg

(299)

C. 160 mg

Rationale:

Step 1: Convert height of the patient to inches:

1 ft/12 inches = 5 ft/x

$x = (5 \times 12)/1 = 60$ inches

60 inches + 10 inches = 70 inches

Step 2: Find the BSA:

$$\text{BSA m}^2 = \sqrt{\frac{([\text{Height (cm)} \times \text{Weight (kg)}])}{3,600}} \text{ or } \sqrt{\frac{([\text{Height (in)} \times \text{Weight (lb)}])}{3,131}}$$

$$\text{BSA} = \sqrt{\frac{([70(\text{in}) \times 180 \ (\text{lb})]) = 2\text{m}^2}{3131}}$$

Step 3: Find out how much medication the patient will receive per dose:

$$\frac{20\text{mg}}{1\text{m}^2} = \frac{x}{2\text{m}^2} \quad x = 40 \text{ mg}$$

Step 4: Find out how much medication the patient will receive per day by multiplying the dose by 4 since the dose is given every 6 hours or 4 times a day:

24/6 = 4

40 mg $\times$ 4 = 160 mg

(299)

A patient with a severe urinary tract infection is ordered 5.5 g of ciprofloxacin to be taken over 14 days. Available at the pharmacy is ciprofloxacin 250 mg tablets. How many tablets should the pharmacy technician dispense for the course of therapy?

A. 22 tablets
B. 11 tablets
C. 308 tablets
D. 45 tablets

(300)

A. 22 tablets

Rationale:

Step 1: Convert the ordered dose to milligrams because the medication is available in mg

1 g/ 1,000 mg = 5.5 g/x

$x = (5.5 \times 1,000)/1 = 5,500$ mg

Hint: When you write proportions, always remember to start with your known, which in this case is the equivalency of 1 g/1,000 mg. Then write your unknown, which in this case is 5.5 g/x.

Also, make sure the units in the known numerator match the units of the unknown numerator and the units in the known denominator match the units in the unknown denominator. If you do not line up your units correctly, you will get a wrong answer.

Another way of writing the proportion is as follows:

1 g/5.5g = 1,000 mg/x

However, you should use only one of the above methods to avoid making mistakes.

Step 2: Figure out how many tablets to dispense using the following formula:

dose ordered ÷ dose available = number of tablets to dispense

So 5,500 mg/250 mg = 22 tablets.

(300)

A patient is ordered 8.4% sodium bicarbonate 150 mEq in 1,000 mL of D₅W to be infused at 100 mL/hr. Sodium bicarbonate is available in 5 mEq/5 mL. How much sodium bicarbonate should be added to the IV bag?

A. 1,786 mL
B. 84 mL
C. 1,000 mL
D. 150 mL

(301)

A patient is ordered 20 mEq of potassium chloride in 1,000 mL of 0.45% NS to be infused over 6 hours using a 10 drops per milliliter infusion set. What is the flow rate of the IV bag in milliliters per hour?

A. 50 mL/hr
B. 167 mL/hr
C. 200 mL/hr
D. 150 mL/hr

(302)

D. 150 mL

Rationale:

Step 1: Figure out how much sodium bicarbonate should be added to the IV bag:

5 mEq/5 mL = 150 mEq/x

x = 150 mL

Hint: Often, word problems will provide more information than you need to find the answer. You should know how to read the problem and how to select the useful information. Sometimes, you will not have to use every number provided.

(301)

B. 167 mL/hr

Rationale:

Step 1: Calculate the infusion rate in milliliters per hour using the following formula:

infusion rate (mL/hr) = total volume to be infused (mL)/total amount of time the IV will run (hr)

infusion rate = 1,000 mL/6 hr = 167 mL/hr

(302)

A patient is ordered 20 mEq of potassium chloride in 1,000 mL of 0.45% NS to be infused over 12 hours using a 10 drops per milliliters infusion set. Potassium chloride is available in a concentration of 2 mEq/mL. What is the flow rate of the IV bag in drops per minute?

A. 14 gtt/min
B. 13 gtt/min
C. 8 gtt/min
D. 6 gtt/min

(303)

A. 14 gtt/min

Rationale:

Step 1: Calculate the infusion rate in milliliters per hour using the following formula:

infusion rate (mL/hr) = total volume to be infused (mL)/total amount of time the IV will run (hr)

infusion rate = 1,000 mL/12 hr = 83 mL/hr

Step 2: Convert the rate to drops per minute using the following formula:

infusion rate (gtt/min) = (infusion rate in mL/hr) (drop factor in gtt/mL) (1 hr/60 min)

infusion rate (gtt/min) = (83 mL/hr) $\times$ (10 gtt/mL) $\times$ (1 hr/60 min) = 13.83 gtt/min = 14 gtt/min

(303)

A cancer patient who weighs 80 kg and is 177 cm in height is ordered Ifosfamide 1.2 gm/m^2/day for 5 consecutive days. How much medication will the patient receive over the course of therapy?

A. 24 mg
B. 5 mg
C. 12 mg
D. 2 mg

(304)

A diabetic patient is ordered 75 units of insulin U-100 in 0.9% NS 100 mL. How many units of insulin should be added to the IV bag?

A. 75 mL
B. 0.75 mL
C. 75,000 mL
D. 0.075 mL

(305)

C. 12 mg

Rationale:

Step 1: Calculate the BSA of the patient:

$$BSA = \sqrt{\frac{weight\ (kg) \times height\ (cm)}{3,600}}$$

BSA = [square root of (80 kg × 177 cm)]/3,600 = 1.98 m²

Step 2: Calculate the medication dose per day:

1.2 gm/m² = x/1.98 m²

x = (1.2 × 1.98)/1 = 2.38 mg

Step 3: Calculate the amount of medication to be given over the course of therapy by multiplying the dose per day by 5:

2.38 mg × 5 = 11.89 mg or 12 mg

(304)

B. 0.75 mL

Rationale:

Insulin U-100 = insulin 100 units/mL so every 1 mL contains 100 units, which means that 75 units will be less than 1 mL.

100 units/mL = 75 units/x

x = 0.75 mL

Hint: The maximum volume that is usually added to an IV bag is 1 mL, though the insulin vial contains 10 mL. Be careful computing because adding 10 mL of insulin to an IV bag can lead to the death of the patient.

(305)

A patient who weighs 135 lb is ordered penicillin G 25,000 units/kg in 100 mL NS every 4 hours for a serious pneumonia infection. How many units will be added to each IV bag?

A. 6 million units
B. 409 units
C. 153,400 units
D. 1.5 million units

(306)

A pharmacy technician receives an order for 1.6 million of penicillin G in 100 mL NS. Penicillin G is diluted to 100,000 units/mL concentration. How many milliliters should be added to the IV bag?

A. 20 mL
B. 0.001 mL
C. 16 mL
D. 62.5 mL

(307)

D. 1.5 million units

Rationale:

Step 1: Convert weight from pounds to kilograms:

1 kg/2.2 lb = x/135 lb

x = 61.36 kg

Step 2: Calculate the dose for the patient:

25,000 units/kg = x/61.36 kg

x = 1,534,000 units or 1.5 million units

(306)

C. 16 mL

Rationale:

100,000 units/mL = 1,600,000 units/x

x = (1,600,000 × 1)/100,000 = 16 mL

(307)

A patient who is 168 lb is ordered dopamine 50 mcg/kg/min to be infused at 400 mg in 250 mL of 0.45% NS using a 60 gtt/mL infusion set. What is the IV flow rate in milliliters per hour?

A. 143 mL/hr
B. 2 mL/hr
C. 315 mL/hr
D. 140 mL/hr

(308)

A. 143 mL/hr

Rationale:

Step 1: Convert weight from pounds to kilograms:

$1\text{ kg}/2.2\text{ lb} = x/168\text{ lb}$

$x = 76.36\text{ kg}$

Step 2: Calculate the dose of medication needed for the patient:

$50\text{ mcg/kg} = x/76.36\text{ kg}$

$x = (50 \times 76.36)/1 = 3{,}818\text{ mcg}$

Step 3: Convert the medication dose from micrograms to milligrams:

$1\text{ mg}/1{,}000\text{ mcg} = x/3{,}818\text{ mcg}$

$x = 3.818\text{ mg or }3.82\text{ mg/min}$

Step 4: Calculate amount of medication the patient will receive in milligrams per hour. To convert from milligrams per minute to milligrams per hour, multiply by 60; to convert from milligrams per hour to milligrams per minute, divide by 60.

$(3.82\text{ mg/min}) \times (60\text{ min}/1\text{ hr}) = 229\text{ mg/hr}$

Step 5: Calculate the amount of medication received by the patient in milliliters per hour:

$400\text{ mg}/250\text{ mL} = 229\text{ mg}/x$

$x = 143\text{ mL or }143\text{ mL/hr}$

(308)

Amoxicillin suspension is diluted using 100 mL of sterile water to a final volume of 150 mL. What is the powder displacement volume?

A. 100 mL
B. 50 mL
C. 250 mL
D. 150 mL

(309)

A patient is ordered labetalol 200 mg in 200 mL of NS to be infused at 2 mg/min using a 60 gtt/mL infusion set. How many milliliters of labetalol will the patient receive per hour?

A. 2 mL
B. 4 mL
C. 60 mL
D. 120 mL

(310)

B. 50 mL

Rationale:

powder displacement volume = final volume − diluent volume

powder volume = 150 mL − 100 mL = 50 mL

(309)

D. 120 mL

Rationale:

Step 1: Figure out how many milliliters the patient is receiving per minute:

$$\frac{200\text{mg}}{200\text{mL}} = \frac{2\text{mg}}{x}$$

$$x = \frac{(200)\times 2}{200} = 2\text{mL per min}$$

Step 2: Figure out how many milliliters per hour the patient is receiving:

$$\frac{2\text{mL}}{1\text{min}} = \frac{x}{60\text{min}}$$

$$x = \frac{(60\times 2)}{1} = 120\text{mL}$$

(310)

A patient is ordered 300 grains of thyroid tablets. Available in the pharmacy is 300 mg tablets of thyroid. How many tablets should be dispensed?

A. 65 tablets
B. 59 tablets
C. 30 tablets
D. 35 tablets

(311)

Dr. White prescribed a patient the following prednisone taper regimen:

- Prednisone 40 mg BID QD for 5 days followed by
- Prednisone 40 mg QD for 5 days followed by
- Prednisone 20 mg QD daily for 11 days

How many 20 mg prednisone tablets should be dispensed?

A. 51 tablets
B. 41 tablets
C. 820 tablets
D. 104 tablets

(312)

A. 65 tablets

Rationale:

Step 1: Convert grains to milligrams:

1 gr = 60 or 65 mg

1 gr/65 mg = 300 gr/x

$x = (300 \times 65)/1 = 19{,}500$ mg

Step 2: Find out how many tablets should be dispensed:

dose ordered ÷ dose available = number of tablets to dispense

19,500 mg/300 mg = 65 tablets

(311)

B. 41 tablets

Rationale:

Step 1: Calculate the total amount of medication the patient would receive:

40 mg × 2 × 5 = 400 mg

40 mg × 1 × 5 = 200 mg

20 mg × 1 × 11 = 220 mg

Total = 400 + 200 + 220 = 820 mg

Step 2: Figure out how many tablets to dispense using the following formula:

dose ordered ÷ dose available = number of tablets to dispense

820 mg ÷ 20 mg = 41 tablets

(312)

Brand name drugs are also known as which of the following?

A. trade
B. proprietary
C. innovator
D. all of the above

(313)

At what temperature are Fahrenheit and Celsius equal?

A. 40°
B. −40°
C. 0°
D. 100°

(314)

D. all of the above

Rationale:

A brand name drug is also known as trade, proprietary, innovator, or pioneer drug. A generic drug would be known as nonproprietary. It can only be produced when the patent for a brand drug expires.

(313)

B. −40°

Rationale:

At −40°, both Fahrenheit and Celsius are the same.

°F = (°C × 1.8) + 32

°F = (−40 × 1.8) + 32 = −40° F

°C = (°F − 32)/1.8

°C = (−40 − 32)/1.8 = −40°C

(314)

Which of the following statements regarding temperature is true?

A. Water boils at 100°F.
B. Body temperature is about 50°C.
C. Room temperature is between 15° and 30°C.
D. Freezing point is about 10°C.

(315)

What is the equivalent of the temperature 86° Celsius in Fahrenheit?

A. 122.8°F
B. 186.8°F
C. 30°F
D. 66°F

(316)

C. Room temperature is between 15° and 30°C.

Rationale:

- Water boils at $100°C = 212°F$.
- Body temperature is about $37°C = 98.6°F$.
- Freezing point is about $0°C = 32°F$.

(315)

B. 186.8°F

Rationale:

- $°F = (°C \times 1.8) + 32$
- $°F = (86 \times 1.8) + 32 = 186.8°F$

(316)

Use Clark's rule to calculate the medication dose for a 12-year-old child who weighs 90 lb if the adult dose is 500 mg.

A. 27 mg
B. 833 mg
C. 250 mg
D. 300 mg

(317)

Use Young's rule to calculate the medication dose for a 12-year-old child who weighs 90 lb if the adult dose is 500 mg.

A. 27 mg
B. 833 mg
C. 250 mg
D. 300 mg

(318)

D. 300 mg

Rationale:

According to Clark's rule:

child's dose = (child's weight in lb × adult dose)/150 lb

child's dose = (90 × 500 mg)/150 lb = 300 mg

Hint: Clark's rule is based on weight and it is the only formula that uses weight in pounds instead of kilograms. In Clark's rule, 150 lb is a constant and so that number never changes.

(317)

C. 250 mg

Rationale:

According to Young's rule:

child dose = age in years/(age + 12) × adult dose

child dose = 12 / (12 + 12) × 500 mg = (12/24) × 500 mg = 250 mg

Hint: Young's rule is preferably used for children between 1 to 12 years of age. Remember that Young's rule is based on age just like *young* refers to age. In Young's rule, 12 is a constant.

(318)

Use Fried's rule to calculate the medication dose for a 6-month-old infant based on the adult dose of 500 mg.

A. 20 mg
B. 167 mg
C. 10 mg
D. 5 mg

(319)

A pharmacy technician receives an order for a child weighing 50 lb whose height is 110 cm. If the adult dose is 250 mg, what is the appropriate child dose?

A. 221 mg
B. 179 mg
C. 83 mg
D. 100 mg

(320)

A. 20 mg

Rationale:

Use Fried's rule:

(child's age in months × adult dose)/150 months = (6 × 500 mg)/150 = 20 mg

Hint: Fried's rule is preferably used for infants up to 2 years of age.

(319)

B. 179 mg

Rationale:

Step 1: Convert weight from pounds to kilograms:

1 kg/2.2 lb = x/50 lb

x = (50 × 1)/2.2 = 22.7 kg

Step 2: Calculate based on the BSA of the child:

$$\text{BSA} = \sqrt{\frac{\text{weight (kg)} \times \text{height (cm)}}{3,600}}$$

BSA = square root of [(50 kg × 110 cm)/3,600] = 1.24 m^2

child's dose = (BSA of child/1.73 m^2) × adult dose

child's dose = (1.24 m^2/1.73 m^2) × 250 mg = 179 mg

Hint: This formula is based on the average adult who weighs 140 lb and has a body surface area of 1.73 m^2.

(320)

A pharmacy technician receives an order for amoxicillin 125 mg q8h × 10 days. Amoxicillin is available in 100 mL bottles with a concentration of 125 mg/5 mL. How many bottles should be dispensed to complete this order?

A. 1.5
B. 1
C. 3
D. 2

(321)

If 600 mg of lidocaine powder is suspended in 150 mL of water, what would be the percent concentration of the suspension?

A. 0.4%
B. 400%
C. 40%
D. 4%

(322)

D. 2

Rationale:

Step 1: Calculate amount of medication needed. Since the concentration of the bottle is 125 mg/5 mL, this indicates that every 5 mL contains 125 mg.

So 5 mL × 3 × 10 = 150 mL.

Step 2: Figure out how many bottles of medication the patient would need. Since each bottle contains 100 mL, 2 bottles should be dispensed. Or you can calculate using the following formula:

dose ordered ÷ dose available = number of bottles to dispense

150 mL/100 mL = 1.5 or 2 bottles

(321)

A. 0.4%

Rationale:

Step 1: Convert from milligrams to grams:

1 g/1,000 mg = x/600 mg

$x = (600 \times 1)/1,000 = 0.6$ g

Step 2: Calculate the percent concentration using the following formula:

$$\text{percent concentration} = \frac{\text{quantity of active ingredient (g or ml)} \times 100}{\text{total quantity (g or ml)}}$$

percent concentration = (0.6 g/150 mL) × 100 = 0.4%

The units of the active and inactive ingredients can only be expressed in grams or milliliters, depending on whether the quantity represents a volume or a solid.

(322)

A patient is ordered metronidazole 500 mg in 100 mL of NS to be infused at a rate of 5 mL/min. Calculate the infusion time.

A. 30 minutes
B. 1 hour
C. 20 minutes
D. 45 minutes

(323)

A patient is ordered potassium chloride 15 mEq in 1,000 mL of 0.45% NS to be infused at a rate of 2 mL/min. How many bags should be dispensed for a 24-hour supply?

A. 1 bag
B. 2 bags
C. 3 bags
D. 4 bags

(324)

C. 20 minutes

Rationale:

Figure out how many minutes it will take for one bag to run out:

infusion time = total volume ÷ rate

So 100 mL ÷ (5 mL/min) = 20 minutes

(323)

C. 3 bags

Rationale:

Step 1: Calculate the infusion time:

infusion time = total volume ÷ rate

1000 mL ÷ (2 mL/min) = 500 minutes (infusion time for each bag)

Step 2: Calculate the amount of IV bags needed for a 24-hour supply. A day is comprised of 24 hours and each hour is 60 minutes, so there is a total of 1,440 minutes per day:

1,000 mL/500 min = x/1,440 minutes; x = (1,440 × 1,000)/500 = 2,880 mL

Step 3: Calculate how many bags should be dispensed:

dose ordered ÷ dose available = amount to be dispensed

2,880 mL ÷ 1,000 mL = 2.88 or 3 bags

(324)

A patient is ordered 30 mEq of potassium chloride in 1,000 mL of 0.45% NS to be infused over 12 hours. Potassium chloride is available in a concentration of 2 mEq/mL. How many milliliters of potassium chloride should be added to each IV bag?

A. 15 mL
B. 30 mL
C. 20 mL
D. 45 mL

(325)

A 6-year-old child with fever was ordered 15 mg/kg of Tylenol 160 mg/5 mL. The child weighs 58 lb. How many teaspoons will the child receive per dose?

A. 1 teaspoon
B. 2 teaspoons
C. 3 teaspoons
D. 2.5 teaspoons

(326)

A. 15 mL

Rationale:

Solve by proportion:

2 mEq/mL = 30 mEq/x

$x = (30 \times 1)/2 = 15$ mL

(325)

D. 2.5 teaspoons

Rationale:

Step 1: Convert pounds to kilograms:

1 kg/2.2 lb = x/58 lb

$x = (58 \times 1)/2.2 = 26.36$ kg

Step 2: Calculate the dose for the child:

15 mg/kg = x/26.36 kg

$x = (26.36 \times 15)/1 = 395$ mg

Step 3: Calculate the dose in milliliters:

160 mg/5 mL = 395 mg/x

$x = (395 \times 5)/160 = 12.4$ mL

Step 4: Convert to teaspoons:

1 tsp/5 mL = x/12.4 mL

$x = 12.4/5 = 2.5$ teaspoons

(326)

How many grams of lidocaine can be found in 20 mL of a lidocaine 2% solution?

A. 0.004 g
B. 0.04 g
C. 0.4 mg
D. 0.4 g

(327)

How many grams of dextrose can be found in 500 mL of $D_{10}W$?

A. 5 g
B. 50 g
C. 500 g
D. 5,000 g

(328)

D. 0.4 g

Rationale:

2 g/100 mL = x/20 mL

x = (2 × 20)/100 = 0.4 g of lidocaine

Hint: 2% = 2 in 100 or 2 g/100 mL

(327)

B. 50 g

Rationale:

$D_{10}W$ = dextrose 10% in water

10% = 10 g dextrose in every 100 mL of water

10 g/100 mL = x/500 mL

x = (500 × 10)/100 = 50 g of dextrose

(328)

Which of the following represents 70% in ratio strength?

A. 1:1
B. 1:2.5
C. 1:3
D. 1:1.43

(329)

Which of the following forms is used to document the destruction of controlled substances?

A. DEA form 222
B. DEA form 106
C. DEA form 41
D. DEA form 224

(330)

D. 1:1.43

Rationale:

70% = 70/100

70/100 = 1/x

$x = (1 \times 100)/70 = 1.43$

So in ratio form, 70% = 1:1.43

To check your work:

$(1/1.43) \times 100 = 70\%$

Hint: When converting to ratio strength, always set the proportion equal to (1/x).

(329)

C. DEA form 41

Rationale:

- DEA form 222 is used for purchasing or returning of expired Schedule II drugs.

- DEA form 106 is used to report lost or stolen controlled substances.

- DEA form 224 is a registration form that enables a pharmacy to dispense controlled substances.

(330)

Which of the following DEA form 222 copies is sent by the supplier to the local DEA?

A. green copy
B. blue copy
C. red copy
D. brown copy

(331)

How many different medication items can be ordered per each DEA form 222?

A. 2
B. 6
C. 8
D. 10

(332)

A. green copy

Rationale:

DEA form 222 is composed of 3 copies as follows:

- Copy 1 (brown) is forwarded to the supplier.

- Copy 2 (green) is forwarded to the supplier and then sent to the DEA.

- Copy 3 (blue) is retained by the purchaser for a minimum of 2 years.

(331)

D. 10

Rationale:

DEA form 222 has 10 lines, and so only 10 items can be ordered per form.

Hint: If a mistake is made while writing a DEA form 222, the form must be voided and kept on file.

(332)

How long is a DEA form 222 valid after its execution by the purchaser?

A. 30 days
B. 60 days
C. 120 days
D. 360 days

(333)

Which of the following DEA forms allows the manufacturing and distribution of controlled substances?

A. DEA form 41
B. DEA form 363
C. DEA form 225
D. DEA form 106

(334)

B. 60 days

Rationale:

A DEA form 222 is no longer valid after 60 days of its execution.

(333)

C. DEA form 225

Rationale:

- DEA form 41 is used to document the destruction of controlled substances.

- DEA form 363 is used for registration of a controlled substance treatment program.

- DEA form 106 is used to report lost or stolen controlled substances.

(334)

Which of the following is the most used reference book in hospital pharmacy?

A. *Red Book*
B. *Orange Book*
C. *Green Book*
D. *Drug Facts and Comparisons*

(335)

A pharmacy technician accidentally spills a hazardous product on the floor of the pharmacy. Which of the following references can be referred to for information on cleanup and disposal of hazardous products?

A. *The Handbook on Injectable Drugs*
B. Safety Data Sheets (SDSs)
C. the *Red Book*
D. the *Physician's Desk Reference (PDR)*

(336)

D. *Drug Facts and Comparisons*

Rationale:

- The *Red Book* is most used in retail pharmacies.

- The *Orange Book* compares therapeutic equivalence of brand and generic drugs.

- There is no such thing as a Green Book.

(335)

B. Safety Data Sheets (SDSs)

Rationale:

- The *Handbook on Injectable Drugs* provides information on compatibility, solubility, and stability of injectable drugs.

- The SDSs provide precautions for safe storage, disposal, handling, and spill cleanup of hazardous materials (HazMat).

- The *Red Book* provides information on the available strengths, sizes, and average wholesale prices (AWP) of drugs.

- The *PDR* is mainly used by physicians. It is a compilation of package inserts of FDA-approved products.

(336)

What is the Orphan Drug Act of 1983?

A. a law that allows the sale of discounted drugs to orphans
B. a law that gives incentives to manufacturers to develop drugs
   for orphaned or rare diseases that affect a small portion of the
   population
C. a law that requires pharmacists to counsel patients taking
   orphaned drugs that are rarely used
D. a law that prohibited adulteration or addition of unlisted
   orphaned ingredients into drug recipes

(337)

Which of the following is not a Schedule III drug?

A. Fioricet
B. hydrocodone and acetaminophen
C. codeine and acetaminophen
D. testosterone

(338)

B. a law that gives incentives to manufacturers to develop drugs for orphaned or rare diseases that affect a small portion of the population

Rationale:

- The Orphan Drug Act of 1983 is legislation that gives incentives to manufacturers to develop drugs for orphaned or rare diseases that affect a small portion of the population.

- The Omnibus Reconciliation Act (OBRA) 1990 requires pharmacists to offer counseling on all new drug prescriptions.

- The Food, Drug, and Cosmetic Act of 1938 indicated that misbranding and adulteration of drugs is illegal. It also required manufacturers to provide package inserts and to follow FDA guidelines to present evidence of safety for new drugs before marketing. This law also gave the FDA authority to issue food standards and inspect factories.

(337)

B. hydrocodone and acetaminophen

Rationale:

As of October 6, 2014, Vicodin (hydrocodone and acetaminophen) was rescheduled from Schedule III to Schedule II.

(338)

Which of the following drugs is a Schedule II drug?

A. cocaine
B. phenobarbital
C. lorazepam
D. marinol

(339)

A. cocaine

Rationale:

Cocaine, which is available in a different formulation than the form found on the streets, may be used in hospitals as a local anesthetic for some eye, ear, and throat surgeries. Phenobarbital is a Schedule IV drug, Lorazepam is a Schedule IV drug, and Marinol is a Schedule III drug.

Hint: Scheduled drugs are habit-forming drugs. They are classified by the DEA into five schedules that range from most highly abused to least likely to be abused:

1. Schedule I drugs are street drugs such as LSD, PSP, heroin, and peyote. These drugs have no medicinal use and are highly abused.

2. Schedule II drugs are highly abused drugs that have medicinal purposes. These include oxycodone, morphine, hydrocodone, cocaine, amphetamines, codeine, Percocet, fentanyl, meperidine, hydromorphone, methylphenidate, Adderall, and secobarbital.

3. Schedule III drugs are less abused than Schedule II drugs. These include Tylenol No. 3, Vicodin, Marinol, testosterone, and cough syrups containing hydrocodone.

4. Schedule IV drugs are comprised of mainly all the benzodiazepines. These also include phentermine, pentazocine, phenobarbital, and diethylpropion.

5. Schedule V drugs or exempt narcotics are the least abused of all the scheduled drugs. These include antitussives with codeine and antidiarrheals with opioids.

(339)

Which of the following organizations enforces the comprehensive drug abuse prevention and control act of 1970?

A. FDA
B. DEA
C. TJC
D. FBI

(340)

A pharmacy technician receives an order for Vicodin i-ii tabs po TID-QID prn × 14d. How many tablets should be dispensed?

A. 42 tablets
B. 56 tablets
C. 112 tablets
D. 168 tablets

(341)

B. DEA

Rationale:

- The FDA is the Food and Drug Administration, which regulates prescription and over-the-counter drugs.

- The DEA is the Drug Enforcement Agency, which deals with controlled substances.

- The TJC is The Joint Commission, which accredits healthcare organizations.

- The FBI is the Federal Bureau of Investigation, which is a governmental agency that investigates crimes.

(340)

C. 112 tablets

Rationale:

Since the patients should have a sufficient supply of the medication, the dose should be calculated using the maximum amount of tablets that may be needed per day.

Step 1: Translate the sig code:

Vicodin i-ii tabs po TID-QID prn $\times$ 14d = Vicodin 1 to 2 tablets orally three to four times a day as needed for 14 days

Step 2: Calculate the maximum amount of tablets a patient may need per day:

Vicodin ii tabs po QID prn = $2 \times 4 = 8$ tablets

Step 3: Calculate the amount of tablets needed for 14 days:

$8 \times 14 = 112$ tablets

(341)

A pharmacy technician received an order for IV gtt OU q3–4h × 7d. How many drops will the patient receive over the course of therapy?

A. 224 drops
B. 168 drops
C. 56 drops
D. 448 drops

(342)

Which of the following abbreviations does not indicate a route of administration?

A. SL
B. SR
C. PR
D. SC

(343)

D. 448 drops

Rationale:

Step 1: Translate the sig code:

IV gtt OU q3–4h × 7d = 4 drops in both eyes every 3–4 hours × 7 days

Step 2: Calculate the maximum amount of drops the patient will need per day:

IV gtt OU q3h = 4 × 2 × 8 = 64 drops

Hint: Every 3 hours = 8 times a day because there are 24 hours a day: 24/3 = 8.

Step 3: Calculate the amount of drops the patient will receive over the course of therapy:

64 drops × 7 days = 448 drops

(342)

B. SR

Rationale:

- SL is the abbreviation for sublingual (under the tongue) route.
- SR is the abbreviation for sustained release, which refers to a drug formulation.
- PR is the abbreviation for per rectum or rectal route.
- SC is the abbreviation for subcutaneous route.

(343)

If a manufacturer markets sugar pills as a cure for headache, which law would the manufacturer violate?

A. Pure Food and Drug Act of 1906
B. Durham Humphrey Act
C. Kefauver-Harris Amendment
D. Food, Drug, and Cosmetic Act of 1938

(344)

A patient who is on captopril for her high blood pressure wants to purchase an OTC cough syrup. You would suspect that:

A. the patient has a cold
B. the patient should be prescribed an antibiotic for her cough
C. the patient may be experiencing an ACE cough and the pharmacist should be alerted
D. none of the above

(345)

D. Food, Drug, and Cosmetic Act of 1938

Rationale:

- The Pure Food and Drug Act of 1906 prohibits the manufacture, sale, or transportation of adulterated or misbranded foods, liquors, and drugs.

- The Durham Humphrey Act distinguished between prescription and over-the-counter drugs prohibiting the sale of legend drugs without a prescription.

- The Kefauver-Harris Amendment requires drugs to be proven pure, safe, and effective.

- The Food, Drug, and Cosmetic Act of 1938 indicated that misbranding and adulteration of drugs is illegal. It also required manufacturers to provide package inserts and to follow FDA guidelines to present evidence of safety for new drugs before marketing. This law also gave the FDA authority to issue food standards and inspect factories.

(344)

C. the patient may be experiencing an ACE cough and the pharmacist should be alerted

Rationale:

Captopril is an ACE inhibitor and cough is one of the most common side effects of ACE inhibitors. The only cure for the cough would be stopping the medication rather than using a cough syrup. The pharmacist would need to be alerted to counsel the patient.

(345)

Digibind is an antidote for which of the following medications?

A. Digoxin
B. vitamin K
C. Coumadin
D. metoprolol

(346)

The remainder of a partial filling for a Schedule II drug must be available for the patient within how many hours?

A. 12
B. 24
C. 48
D. 72

(347)

A. digoxin

Rationale:

- Digibind is the antidote for digoxin toxicity.

- Vitamin K is the antidote for Coumadin.

(346)

D. 72

Rationale:

The remainder of a partial filling must be available for the patient within 72 hours or the prescription would be voided and a new prescription order would be needed.

However, Schedule II drugs for long-term care facilities and terminally ill patients can be partially filled for up to 60 days.

(347)

Which of the following healthcare professionals may not take a telephone order from a physician?

A. pharmacy technician
B. registered nurse
C. pharmacist
D. respiratory therapist

(348)

Which of the following sig codes indicates that a medication should be taken after a meal?

A. AC
B. PC
C. QD
D. AD

(349)

A. pharmacy technician

Rationale:

Authorized healthcare professionals who may receive physician telephone orders include registered nurses, pharmacists, and respiratory therapists. However, pharmacy technicians are not authorized to receive telephone orders.

(348)

B. PC

Rationale:

- AC = before a meal
- PC = after a meal
- QD = daily or every day
- AD = right ear

Hint: To remember that AC means before a meal and PC is after a meal, remember that A comes before C in the alphabet.

(349)

Which of the following is not true regarding the Poison Prevention Packaging Act of 1970?

A. It requires most drugs to be packaged in child-resistant packages to prevent accidental child poisoning.

B. Exceptions to the law include oral medicines and controlled substances.

C. A patient may sign a release form to waive the right for childproof packaging.

D. Drugs dispensed in an institution may not require childproof packaging.

(350)

The Combat Methamphetamine Epidemic Act of 2005 regulated which of these drugs behind the counter?

A. ephedrine

B. pseudoephedrine

C. phenylpropanolamine

D. all of the above

(351)

B. Exceptions to the law include oral medicines and controlled substances.

Rationale:

Exceptions to the law include nitroglycerin sublingual, sublingual and chewable forms of isosorbide dinitrate in 10 mg or less, erythromycin ethylsuccinate in packages containing not more than 16 g, potassium supplements in packets containing not more than 50 mEq per dose, pancrelipase preparations, and anhydrous cholestyramine in powder form.

(350)

D. all of the above

Rationale:

All of the options provided are regulated by the Combat Methamphetamine Epidemic Act. The law was created to stop the illegal production of crystal meth. It prohibits the sale of more than 3.6 g of the methamphetamine products for each customer per day and limits sale to 9 g per 30 days.

A log book must be kept with each customer's name, address, date and time of purchase, name of drug, quantity sold, and signature of customer. Also, the customer must present the pharmacy with a photo ID.

(351)

Once an investigational study is complete, what happens to the remaining drugs?

A. They are kept by the pharmacy in case another patient needs them.
B. They are destroyed and recorded on a destruction log.
C. They are given to the patient to continue the therapy at home.
D. They are returned to the sponsor along with the record logs.

(352)

Which of the following healthcare professionals cannot prescribe medications?

A. nurse practitioner
B. physician assistant
C. podiatrist
D. chiropractor

(353)

D. they are returned to the sponsor along with the record logs

Rationale:

Investigational drugs can only be ordered by a physician. They must be stored in the pharmacy in a separate area away from other drugs. The pharmacy must keep a dispensing log and a perpetual inventory of the investigational drugs on hand to ensure that the drugs are not diverted.

(352)

D. chiropractor

Rationale:

Chiropractors are not licensed to prescribe medications.

(353)

Which of the following drug classes should be avoided while on enoxaparin (Lovenox), warfarin (Coumadin), and clopidogrel (Plavix)?

A. NSAIDs
B. macrolides
C. antihistamines
D. proton pump inhibitors

(354)

Which of the following is not a side effect of anticholinergic agents?

A. dry mouth
B. constipation
C. excessive urination
D. blurred vision

(355)

A. NSAIDs

Rationale:

NSAIDs (nonsteroidal anti-inflammatory drugs) should not be taken with anticoagulants or antiplatelets. Concomitant use may lead to hemorrhage.

(354)

C. excessive urination

Rationale:

Excessive urination is not a side effect of anticholinergic agents. Anticholinergic side effects include dry mouth, drowsiness, dizziness, nausea and vomiting, restlessness or moodiness (in some children), lack of urination, blurred vision, and confusion.

Anticholinergic agents or cholinergic antagonists (blockers) have drying effects on secretions and so they are used to treat cold and allergy symptoms, excessive urination, GI distress, and mydriasis (dilation of the pupil).

(355)

Which of the following is not a side effect of cholinergic agents?

A. hypertension
B. diarrhea
C. excessive urination
D. sweating or flushing

(356)

Which of the following is an effective antidote to episodes of hypoglycemia?

A. Glucotrol
B. glyburide
C. glucagon
D. Glucophage

(357)

A. hypertension

Rationale:

Cholinergic side effects include hypotension (low blood pressure), low heart rate, diarrhea, sweating or flushing, miosis (constriction of the pupil), and breathing difficulty.

Cholinergic agents act on those receptors in which acetylcholine acts as the major neurotransmitter that activates the receptor.

(356)

C. glucagon

Rationale:

Glucagon is an effective antidote against hypoglycemia. Glucotrol, glyburide, and Glucophage are oral antidiabetics effective against type 2 diabetes.

(357)

Which of the following drug classes is a medication that thins the mucus so it may be easier to expel from the chest?

A. expectorant
B. antitussive
C. decongestant
D. antiseptic

(358)

Which of the following is not a side effect of alpha-adrenergic agonist agents?

A. vasoconstriction
B. rebound congestion
C. low blood pressure or hypotension
D. tremors

(359)

A. expectorant

Rationale:

- An expectorant thins the mucus so it may be easier to expel from the chest. An example is Robitussin.

- An antitussive exhibits cough suppressant effects and is usually recommended for dry or nonproductive coughs caused by colds, flu, or lung infections. An example is dextromethorphan (DM).

- A decongestant relieves nasal congestion by causing vasoconstriction. An example is pseudoephedrine.

- An antiseptic can inhibit the growth of microorganisms and is usually a topical agent. Examples include iodine and chlorhexidine gluconate.

(358)

C. low blood pressure or hypotension

Rationale:

Alpha-adrenergic agonist agents are used as vasopressors, nasal decongestants, and eye decongestants.

The side effects include vasoconstriction, elevated blood pressure, rebound congestion, and tremors.

(359)

If an emergency Schedule II drug is ordered by a physician, a written order must be submitted to the pharmacy within how much time?

A. 4 hours after calling in the order
B. 24 hours after calling in the order
C. 48 hours after calling in the order
D. 7 days after calling in the order

(360)

D. 7 days

Rationale:

In cases of extreme emergency, a pharmacy may fill a limited amount of a Schedule II order without a prescription. However, the physician must submit a written order to the pharmacy within 1 week. If the order is not received by the pharmacy within the 1-week timeframe, the DEA must be informed of the transaction.

(360)

Determine which of the following DEA numbers are valid for Dr. Rachel White.

A. AW5436789
B. BW5448899
C. AW6789450
D. both B and C

(361)

D. both B and C

Rationale:

The first letter of the DEA number depends on the registrant type. It could be an "A" if the registrant is an older entity; a "B" if it is a hospital/clinic; a "C" if it is a practitioner; a "D" if it is a teaching institution; an "E" if it is a manufacturer; an "F" if it is a distributor; a "G" if it is a researcher; an "H" if it is an analytical lab; a "J" if it is an importer; a "K" for an exporter; an "L" for a reverse distributor; an "M" for a mid-level practitioner (example: nurse practitioner, PA); and "N-U" for narcotic treatment programs.

The second letter is usually the first letter of the doctor's last name. In this case, "W" is correct.

The two letters are followed by seven digits that have a mathematical relationship as follows:

1. Add the first, third, and fifth digits:

    $5 + 3 + 7 = 15$

2. Add the second, fourth and sixth digit and then multiply the sum by 2:

    $(4 + 6 + 8) \times 2 = 36$

3. Add the sum of the answers from step 1 and step 2:

    $36 + 15 = 51$

4. If the last digit of the DEA number matches the last digit of the above sum, then the DEA number is valid. If the number is different, it is an invalid DEA.

In this case, AW5436789 is invalid.

(361)

Which of the following elements of a prescription is not generally required?

A. Patient name
B. Home address
C. Indication
D. Drug strength

(362)

C. Indication

Rationale:

The following are important elements of a prescription:

- Name and home address of patient
- Date prescription was written
- Drug name, dosage form, drug strength, and total quantity
- Directions for use, route of administration, frequency, and duration of use
- Quantity to be dispensed
- Number of refills
- Substitution directive (if needed)
- Signature of the prescriber
- DEA number if controlled substance is prescribed

(362)

Which of the following is a correct way of cleaning the laminar airflow hood?

A. Clean the laminar airflow hood surface, side walls, and the hanging rack with lint-free absorbent cloth first with sterile water followed by 70% isopropyl alcohol using a side-to-side and a front-to-back motion.

B. Spray all surfaces with 70% isopropyl alcohol. Wipe down the HEPA filter first, followed by the work surface, side walls, and the hanging rack using a side-to-side and a back-to-front motion.

C. Clean the laminar airflow hood surface, side walls, and the hanging rack with lint-free absorbent cloth first with sterile water followed by 70% isopropyl alcohol using a side-to-side and a back-to-front motion.

D. Clean the laminar airflow hood surface, side walls, and the hanging rack with gauze pads first with bleach followed by 70% isopropyl alcohol using a side-to-side and a back-to-front motion.

(363)

How many milliliters are contained in 2 pints of liquid?

A. 946 mL
B. 1892 mL
C. 454 mL
D. 60 mL

(364)

C. Clean the laminar airflow hood surface, side walls, and the hanging rack with lint-free absorbent cloth first with sterile water followed by 70% isopropyl alcohol using a side-to-side and a back-to-front motion.

Rationale:

The laminar airflow hood must be cleaned with lint-free absorbent cloth first with sterile water followed by 70% isopropyl alcohol using a side-to-side and a back-to-front motion. The surface of the hood should be wiped from the inside out using a broad side-to-side motion.

Alcohol should not be sprayed on surfaces and it should not come in direct contact with the HEPA filter because it could damage it.

After cleaning the hood, the compounder must wait 30 minutes before using it.

(363)

A. 946 mL

Rationale:

1 pint = 473 mL

2 pints = 946 mL

(364)

What is another name for vitamin B$_9$?

A. cyanocobalamin
B. thiamine
C. folic acid
D. pyridoxine

(365)

Which of the following drugs would precipitate if mixed with calcium gluconate?

A. magnesium sulfate
B. sodium chloride
C. potassium chloride
D. potassium phosphate

(366)

C. folic acid

Rationale:

- Vitamin B_1 = thiamine
- Vitamin B_2 = riboflavin
- Vitamin B_3 = niacin
- Vitamin B_5 = pantothenic acid
- Vitamin B_6 = pyridoxine
- Vitamin B_9 = folic acid
- Vitamin B_{12} = cyanocobalamin

(365)

D. potassium phosphate

Rationale:

When mixing parenteral nutrition solutions, potassium phosphate and calcium gluconate should not be added one after the other due to incompatibility. Usually, potassium phosphate is added first and then calcium gluconate at the very end after all other electrolytes are added.

(366)

Which of the following DAW codes indicates that drug substitution is allowed because the generic drug is not available in the pharmacy?

A. 4
B. 5
C. 6
D. 7

(367)

A. 4

Rationale:

Dispense as written (DAW) codes are as follows:

- DAW 0 = no DAW specified
- DAW 1 = brand name requested by physician (substitution allowed)
- DAW 2 = brand name requested by patient (substitution allowed)
- DAW 3 = brand name selected by pharmacist (substitution allowed)
- DAW 4 = generic is not available in the pharmacy (substitution allowed)
- DAW 5 = brand name is dispensed and priced as generic (substitution allowed)
- DAW 6 = override
- DAW 7 = brand name mandated by law (substitution not allowed)
- DAW 8 = generic drug backordered in marketplace (substitution allowed)
- DAW 9 = other

These codes can affect payment of claims.

(367)

The total cost of Lovenox 40 mg at Joe's pharmacy is $3,000 for 24 injections. If the pharmacy sells products at AWP + 20% markup + $5 dispensing fee, what is the average wholesale price (AWP) of one injection?

A. $125
B. $155
C. $95
D. $144

(368)

C. $95

Rationale:

Step 1: Calculate the cost of one injection:

$3,000/24 injections = x/1 injection

$x = (3,000 \times 1)/24 = $125 per injection

Step 2: Calculate the average wholesale price:

total cost = AWP + 20% markup + $5 dispensing fee

AWP = total cost − 20% markup − $5 dispensing fee

markup = 20/100 × ($125) = $25

AWP = $125 − $25 − $5 = $95 per injection

(368)

Which of the following is a term used to denote directions for a patient?

A. superscription
B. inscription
C. signa
D. subscription

(369)

What does the abbreviation HIPAA stand for?

A. heparin-induced platelet activation assay
B. High Individual Privacy and Accountability Act
C. Health Insurance Portability and Accountability Act
D. Health Information Protecting and Accounting Act

(370)

C. signa

Rationale:

- Superscription includes the prescription date, patient name, patient address, patient age, and the symbol Rx, which means "recipe" or "to receive."

- Inscription is the part of the prescription that includes the name and amount of the medication prescribed or strength of each ingredient.

- Subscription refers to the instructions to the pharmacist, which usually includes the total quantity to be dispensed.

(369)

C. Health Insurance Portability and Accountability Act

Rationale:

HIPAA stands for Health Insurance Portability and Accountability Act.

(370)

How many pounds are there in 36 ounces?

A. 3 lb
B. 2.5 lb
C. 2.25 lb
D. 1.5 lb

(371)

A certified pharmacy technician can perform which of the following duties?

A. drug utilization review (DUR)
B. contact prescribers regarding drug therapy modification
C. perform dispensing process validation
D. with the approval of the pharmacist, transfer prescriptions issued for nonscheduled drugs between pharmacies

(372)

C. 2.25 lb

Rationale:

1 lb = 16 oz

So 1 lb/16 oz = x/36 oz

$x = (1 \times 36)/16 = 2.25$ lb

(371)

D. with the approval of the pharmacist, transfer prescriptions issued for nonscheduled drugs between pharmacies

Rationale:

A pharmacy technician cannot perform DURs, contact prescribers regarding drug therapy modification, and perform dispensing process validation. However, a pharmacy technician can transfer nonscheduled drug prescriptions between pharmacies with pharmacist approval.

(372)

How many times can Schedule III–V controlled substances be transferred between pharmacies?

A. 10
B. 5
C. 3
D. 1

(373)

A nuclear pharmacy technician must have access to which of the following equipment?

A. body and ring dose meters
B. protective clothing
C. decontamination kit
D. all of the above

(374)

D. 1

Rationale:

According to DEA rules, Schedule III–V controlled substances can only be transferred once between pharmacies. However, pharmacies with electronically linked databases can transfer prescriptions for Schedules III–V an infinite amount of times. Schedule II drugs cannot be transferred.

(373)

D. all of the above

Rationale:

Body and ring dose meters, protective clothing, and a decontamination kit are all needed equipment that a nuclear pharmacy technician must have access to.

(374)

A pharmacy receives an order for a Persantine IV bag for a stress test. Persantine is a radiopharmaceutical dosed at 0.57 mg/kg. How many mg should be added to an IV bag for a patient who weighs 180 lb?

A. 46.6 mg
B. 143.5 mg
C. 694.7 mg
D. 225.7 mg

(375)

Which of the following auxiliary labels should be affixed to containers of anti-infective agents?

A. take with dairy products
B. avoid dairy products
C. finish all this medication unless otherwise directed by the prescriber
D. may cause drowsiness

(376)

A. 46.6 mg

Rationale:

Step 1: Convert pounds to kilograms:

1 kg/2.2 lb = x/180 lb

$x = (180 \times 1)/2.2 = 81.82$ kg

Step 2: Calculate the dose for the patient:

0.57 mg/kg = x/81.82 kg

$x = (81.82 \times 0.57)/1 = 46.6$ mg

(375)

C. finish all this medication unless otherwise directed by the prescriber

Rationale:

Anti-infective agents include antibiotic, antiviral, and antifungal medications. These medications should be completed unless otherwise directed by the prescriber to avoid the development of resistance.

(376)

Which of the following auxiliary labels should be affixed to containers of suspension antibiotics?

A. refrigerate
B. shake well
C. may cause drowsiness
D. both A and B

(377)

Which of the following auxiliary labels should be affixed to containers of narcotics, muscle relaxants, and antihypertensive agents?

A. may cause drowsiness
B. take on an empty stomach
C. do not drink with alcohol
D. both A and C

(378)

D. both A and B

Rationale:

Suspension antibiotics should be refrigerated and shaken well. Most have a stability limit of 14 days unless otherwise indicated by the manufacturer.

(377)

D. both A and C

Rationale:

Narcotics, muscle relaxants, and antihypertensive agents may cause drowsiness and dizziness. These effects may be intensified by alcohol.

(378)

Which of the following medications can alter the effectiveness of birth control?

A. antibiotics
B. benzodiazepines
C. NSAIDs
D. muscle relaxants

(379)

Which of the following auxiliary labels should be affixed to containers of sulfonamides, fluoroquinolones, and tetracyclines?

A. may cause drowsiness
B. take on an empty stomach
C. may cause photosensitivity
D. do not drink with alcohol

(380)

A. antibiotics

Rationale:

Antibiotics can reduce the absorption and metabolism of birth control. As a result, another method of pregnancy prevention is required while on antibiotics.

(379)

C. may cause photosensitivity

Rationale:

- Sulfonamides, fluoroquinolones, and tetracyclines may cause photosensitivity. Prolonged exposure to sunlight should be avoided while on these medications.

- Tetracycline agents should be taken on an empty stomach except for minocycline, doxycycline, and instances of long-term use of tetracyclines.

- Tetracyclines and fluoroquinolones should not be taken within 1 hour of ingesting dairy products, antacids, or iron preparations.

- Sulfonamides should be taken with plenty of water.

(380)

Which of the following fruits and fruit juices should be avoided while on calcium channel blockers and HMG-CoA enzyme inhibitors?

A. strawberry
B. orange
C. grapefruit
D. pineapple

(381)

Which of the following statements is true regarding the herbal supplement chamomile?

A. It may interfere with the efficacy of hormonal therapies.
B. It may cause additive effects and side effects when used along with benzodiazepines.
C. It may reduce the effectiveness of birth control pills.
D. all of the above

(382)

C. grapefruit

Rationale:

Grapefruit and grapefruit juices should be avoided while on calcium channel blockers and HMG-CoA enzyme inhibitors (statins). Exceptions include rosuvastatin, diltiazem, and amlodipine.

(381)

D. all of the above

Rationale:

Chamomile may interfere with the efficacy of hormonal therapies, cause additive effects and side effects when used concurrently with benzodiazepines, and reduce the effectiveness of birth control pills. In addition, chamomile can interact with warfarin, which leads to increased effects resulting in overdose and hemorrhage. It can also cause additive effects and side effects when given concurrently with buccal fentanyl.

(382)

What is the route of administration for lozenges and troches?

A. oral
B. buccal
C. transdermal
D. rectal

(383)

Which of the following drugs require the distribution of a package insert to the patient?

A. accutane
B. birth control pills
C. metered dose inhalers
D. all of the above

(384)

B. buccal

Rationale:

Lozenges and troches are administered through the buccal route or oral transmucosa. This indicates that they are placed between the gum and inner cheek until they dissolve and get absorbed through the oral mucosal membranes.

(383)

D. all of the above

Rationale:

Federal law requires the distribution of a package insert to the patient with the following drugs: Accutane, birth control pills, metered dose inhalers, and agents that contain estrogen or progesterone.

(384)

Which of the following drugs requires weekly complete blood cell counts (CBCs) prior to drug dispensing?

A. clozapine
B. Prozac
C. paroxetine
D. sertraline

(385)

Which of the following auxiliary labels should be affixed to containers of NSAIDs?

I.   Take with food.
II. Take with plenty of water.
III. May cause photosensitivity.
IV. Do not refrigerate.
    A. I and II only
    B. I and III only
    C. II and III only
    D. II and IV only

(386)

A. clozapine

Rationale:

Clozapine is an antipsychotic drug that may lead to agranulocytosis. In 1990, the "no blood, no drug" program was initiated, which required weekly CBCs prior to drug dispensing of clozapine (Clozaril). Prozac, paroxetine, and sertraline are SSRIs.

(385)

A. I and II only

Rationale:

Most NSAIDs have to be taken with food and plenty of water to prevent GI upset unless otherwise indicated by the manufacturer.

(386)

Which of the following auxiliary labels should be affixed to containers of cytotoxic agents?

A. may cause drowsiness
B. antineoplastic material—handle properly
C. shake well
D. may be habit-forming

(387)

Which of the following drug classes are considered vesicants?

A. antitumor antibiotics
B. mechlorethamine
C. vinca alkaloids
D. all of the above

(388)

B. antineoplastic material—handle properly

Rationale:

Containers of cytotoxic agents should be affixed with the auxiliary label: Antineoplastic material—Handle properly.

(387)

D. all of the above

Rationale:

Vesicants can cause severe skin blistering in addition to eye and mucosal pain and irritation. Many chemotherapy drugs are considered vesicants. These agents include antitumor antibiotics (doxorubicin, daunorubicin, mitomycin, idarubicin, epirubicin, and actinomycin), mechlorethamine, vinca alkaloids (vinblastine, vinorelbine, and vincristine), taxanes (paclitaxel [Abraxane], docetaxel), and many others (amsacrine, etoposide, streptozocin, oxaliplatin, and ifosfamide).

(388)

How many milliliters are in a cup?

A. 120 mL
B. 240 mL
C. 360 mL
D. 480 mL

(389)

B. 240 mL

Rationale:

1 cup = 8 ounces and each 1 ounce = 30 mL

1 ounce/30 mL = 8 ounces/x

$x = (8 \times 30)/1 = 240$ mL

Here are some other important conversions to remember:

Measure	Equivalent
1 teaspoon	5 mL
1 tablespoon	15 mL or 3 teaspoons
4 mL	1 dram
1 fluid ounce	30 mL
1 ounce (solid)	30 g
1 cup	8 ounces
1 quart	946 mL = 2 pints
1 pint	2 cups = 16 ounces = 480 mL or 473 mL (exact)
1 gallon	4 quarts = 3,785 mL
1 kg	2.2 lb
1 grain	60 or 65 mg
1 lb	454 g
1 drop	20 mL

(389)

Which of the following statements regarding temperature is NOT true?

A. Water boils at 100°F.
B. Body temperature is about 37°C.
C. Refrigerator temperature is between 2° and 8°C.
D. Freezer temperature is between −20° and −26°C.

(390)

Who decides if a new drug on the market should be added to the hospital's drug formulary?

A. the doctors on staff
B. the pharmacy director
C. the nursing supervisors
D. the pharmacy and therapeutic (P & T) committee

(391)

A. Water boils at 100°F.

Rationale:

Water boils at 100°C = 212°F.

Body temperature is about 37°C = 98.6°F.

Refrigerator temperature is between 2° and 8°C = 36° and 46°F.

Freezer temperature is between −20° and −26°C = −4° and −14°F.

(390)

D. the pharmacy and therapeutics (P & T) committee

Rationale:

The pharmacy and therapeutics (P & T) committee is composed of physicians, pharmacists, and other health professionals who meet monthly to discuss any matters pertaining to the drug formulary, nonformulary drugs, and investigational drugs. This includes discussions of drug use, cost effectiveness, institutional compliance, distribution, administration, and prescribing of drugs within the institution.

(391)

Which of the following drugs is an antifungal medication?

A. omeprazole
B. miconazole
C. lansoprazole
D. pantoprazole

(392)

Which of the following is an antihypertensive drug class?

A. ACE inhibitors
B. angiotensin II receptor blockers
C. beta blockers
D. all of the above

(393)

B. miconazole

Rationale:

Miconazole is an antifungal medication. Omeprazole, lansoprazole, and pantoprazole are proton pump inhibitors recommended for heartburn. Most antifungal medications end with the suffix *-conazole*. Examples include fluconazole, itraconazole, and ketoconazole.

(392)

D. all of the above

Rationale:

Antihypertensive drug classes include ACE inhibitors, alpha blockers, alpha-beta blockers, angiotensin II reuptake blockers, beta blockers, calcium channel blockers, diuretics, nervous system inhibitors, and vasodilators. These are drug classes that lower blood pressure.

(393)

A 58-year-old patient is prescribed morphine sulfate CR 15 mg tablets following major surgery. He comes to the pharmacy for a refill 1 week after his medication was originally filled and indicates that he misplaced the container of medication and he is in severe pain. Which of the following would be the most appropriate action to take as a pharmacy technician?

A. Advise the patient that he cannot obtain a refill unless he receives a new prescription from his physician.
B. Fill a limited emergency dose for the patient to take care of his pain.
C. Fill the prescription and advise the patient that he needs to call his physician to fax a refill order to the pharmacy.
D. none of the above

(394)

A pharmacy technician receives a written prescription that reads: Cortisporin otic ii drops AD TID × 2–3 days. Which of the following is the appropriate route of administration?

A. eye
B. ear
C. orally after meals
D. intradermally

(395)

A. Advise the patient that he cannot obtain a refill unless he receives a new prescription from his physician.

Rationale:

Morphine sulfate controlled release (CR) or MS-Contin is a Schedule II narcotic and cannot be refilled. The patient must get a new prescription from the physician.

(394)

B. ear

Rationale:

Otic is the medical term for "ear."

(395)

A pharmacy technician receives a written prescription that reads: ii gtt AD TID × 2–3 days. Which of the following is the correct translation?

A. Instill 2 drops into the left ear three times per day for 2 to 3 days.
B. Instill 2 drops into the right ear three times per day for 2 to 3 days.
C. Instill 2 drops into the left eye three times per day for 2 to 3 days.
D. Instill 2 drops into the right eye three times per day for 2 to 3 days.

(396)

A pharmacy technician receives a written prescription that reads: Moxifloxacin 0.5% iii gtt OU TID × 7d. If each bottle has a total volume of 5 mL, how many bottles should be dispensed to complete this therapy?

A. 1
B. 2
C. 7
D. 8

(397)

B. Instill 2 drops into the right ear three times per day for 2 to 3 days.

Rationale:

ii = 2

gtt = drops

AD = right ear

TID = three times per day

(396)

B. 2

Rationale:

Step 1: Calculate the amount of drops needed over the course of the therapy:

iii gtt OU TID × 7d = 3 × 2 × 3 × 7 = 126 drops

Step 2: Convert the drops to milliliters:

1 mL = 16 drops

1 mL/16 drops = x/126 drops

$x = (1 \times 126)/16 = 7.875$ mL = 7.9 mL or 8 mL

Step 3: Figure out how many bottles need to be dispensed. Since each bottle is 5 mL, 2 bottles would need to be dispensed to fill the order.

Or use the following formula:

dose ordered ÷ dose available = number of items to dispense

8 mL ÷ 5 mL = 1.6 or 2 bottles

(397)

A diabetic patient is ordered 5 units of regular insulin before every meal and 40 units of Lantus insulin QHS. How many vials of Lantus insulin will the patient need over the course of 1 month?

A. 1
B. 2
C. 3
D. 4

(398)

Which of the following information is not necessary in determining the status of a patient's insurance coverage?

A. gender
B. marital status
C. food preferences
D. the name of the drug plan and identifying numbers

(399)

B. 2

Rationale:

Step 1: Calculate how many milliliters of insulin Lantus the patient needs per day:

1 mL/100 units $= x$/40 units

$x = (1 \times 40)/100 = 0.4$ mL

Step 2: Calculate the amount of insulin needed per month:

0.4 mL $\times$ 30 $= 12$ mL

Step 3: Figure out how many vials the patient would need:

dose ordered $\div$ dose available $=$ number of items to dispense

12 mL $\div$ 10 mL $= 1.2$ or 2 vials

Hint: Each vial of insulin is 10 mL; therefore, the dose available is equal to 10 mL.

So the concentration of insulin Lantus is U-100 or 100 units per milliliter.

(398)

C. food preferences

Rationale:

The necessary information for determining insurance coverage of a patient include full name, gender, marital status, birth date, home address and telephone number, name of any and all drug plans and identifying numbers, plan policyholder's name and relation to the patient, and any food and drug allergies.

(399)

Which of the following is part of the adjudication process?

I. Determination of patient drug coverage eligibility
II. Lowering patient payments
III. Determination of patient copayment
IV. Determination of reimbursement amount to the pharmacy
   A. I, II, and III only
   B. I, II, and IV only
   C. I, III, and IV only
   D. II, III, and IV only

(400)

Which of the following is not a patient's protected health information (PHI)?

A. name
B. address
C. telephone number
D. eye color

(401)

C. I, III, and IV only

Rationale:

The adjudication process includes the following:

- Determination of patient drug coverage eligibility
- Determination of patient copayment
- Determination of reimbursement amount to the pharmacy

(400)

D. eye color

Rationale:

PHIs include the patient's name, address, name of relatives and employers, marital status, birth date, telephone numbers, fax number, e-mail address, social security number, medical and or pharmacy record number, health plan beneficiary number, account number, certificate or license number, serial number of any vehicle or other device, website address, fingerprints or voiceprints, and photographic images.

(401)

What does the NCPDP ID identify?

A. the insurance provider
B. the patient
C. the pharmacy
D. the prescriber

(402)

Which of the following statements is true regarding the notice of privacy practices (NPP)?

A. It discloses the patient's rights.
B. It is given to patients at their first visit to a doctor's office or pharmacy.
C. It explains how patient PHIs may be used.
D. all of the above

(403)

C. the pharmacy

Rationale:

The national council for prescription drug programs (NCPDP) provider identification number is a seven-digit unique pharmacy identification number used during claim processing.

(402)

D. all of the above

Rationale:

The notice of privacy practices (NPP) describes to the patients their rights and how their PHIs may be used. It is given to patients at their first visit to a doctor's office or pharmacy.

(403)

Patients' right to confidentiality in healthcare-related practices is primarily protected by which of the following laws?

A. discretionary law
B. HIPAA privacy rule
C. compliance rules
D. standard code of ethics

(404)

Which of the following would be responsible for managing pharmacy benefits?

A. PBM
B. MAC
C. AWP
D. ATM

(405)

B. HIPAA privacy rule

Rationale:

The HIPAA privacy rule ensures patients' right to confidentiality in healthcare-related practices.

(404)

A. PBM

Rationale:

- A pharmacy benefits manager (PBM) administers pharmacy benefits for third-party payers (insurances).

- The maximum allowable cost (MAC) is an insurance reimbursement formula based on the lowest available cost of the generic equivalent to the drug prescribed.

- The average wholesale price (AWP) is the average wholesale cost of a drug before the addition of markups and dispensing fees.

- An ATM is an automatic teller machine, which is irrelevant to this topic.

(405)

How much dextrose 70% should be mixed with dextrose 20% to make 400 mL of a 30% dextrose solution?

A. 320 mL of the 70% dextrose and 80 mL of the 20% dextrose
B. 80 mL of the 70% dextrose and 320 mL of the 20% dextrose
C. 100 mL of the 70% dextrose and 300 mL of the 20% dextrose
D. 300 mL of the 70% dextrose and 100 mL of the 20% dextrose

(406)

B. 80 mL of the 70% dextrose and 320 mL of the 20% dextrose

Rationale:

Step 1: This is an alligation problem. Draw a grid similar to a tic-tac-toe grid and fill it out as follows:

1. Record the desired percentage or the percentage of the final solution that you are making in the middle.

2. Record the higher of the two concentrations that you are mixing together in the upper left-hand corner box.

3. Record the lower of the two concentrations that you are mixing together in the lower left-hand corner box.

4. Subtract the numbers from the desired concentration and record the results in the respective diagonal boxes:

     70% − 30% = 40 parts

     30% − 20% = 10 parts

70%		10 parts
	30%	
20%		40 parts

10 parts out of the 70% dextrose are needed and

40 parts out of the 20% dextrose

Total parts = 10 + 40 = 50 parts

Step 2: Calculate the amount of dextrose needed of each concentration:

10 parts/50 parts = x/400 mL x = (10 × 400)/50 = 80 mL of the 70% dextrose

40 parts/50 parts = x/400 mL

x = (40 × 400)/50 = 320 mL of the 20% dextrose

Hint: To check your work, add up the sum of the two portions and it should equal the final volume. For this case: 320 mL + 80 mL = 400 mL.

(406)

How much dextrose 70% should be mixed with 500 mL of dextrose 10% to make a 45% dextrose solution?

A. 292 mL of the 70% dextrose
B. 857 mL of the 70% dextrose
C. 700 mL of the 70% dextrose
D. 1,200 mL of the 70% dextrose

(407)

C. 700 mL of the 70% dextrose

Rationale:

Step 1: This is an alligation problem. Draw a grid similar to a tic-tac-toe grid and fill it out as follows:

1. Record the desired percentage or the percentage of the final solution that you are making in the middle.

2. Record the higher of the two concentrations that you are mixing together in the upper left-hand corner box.

3. Record the lower of the two concentrations that you are mixing together in the lower left-hand corner box.

4. Subtract the numbers from the desired concentration and record the results in the respective diagonal boxes:

$70\% - 45\% = 25$ parts

$45\% - 10\% = 35$ parts

70%		35 parts
	45%	
10%		25 parts

35 parts out of the 70% dextrose is needed and

25 parts out of the 10% dextrose or $35:25 = 7:5$

Total parts $= 7 + 5 = 12$ parts

Step 2: Calculate the amount of 70% dextrose needed:

7 parts/5 parts $= x/500$ mL

$x = (7 \times 500)/5 = 700$ mL of the 70% dextrose

(407)

If a patient receives 5 mL of a 20% solution, how many milligrams of the solution did he receive?

A. 1,000 mg
B. 400 mg
C. 25 mg
D. 1 mg

(408)

A. 1,000 mg

Rationale:

20% = 20 g/100 mL

20 g/100 mL = x/5 mL

$x = (20 \times 5)/100 = 1$ g = 1,000 mg

(408)

A pharmacy technician is asked to dilute 300 mL of a 50% solution of acetic acid to a 20% concentration. How much diluent should be added?

A. 750 mL
B. 450 mL
C. 120 mL
D. 180 mL

(409)

B. 450 mL

Rationale:

Step 1: Use the dilution equation:

concentration 1 (C1) × quantity 1 (Q1) = concentration 2 (C2) × quantity 2 (Q2)

50% × (300 mL) = 20% × (x)

$x = (50 × 300)/20 = 750$ mL

Step 2: Calculate the amount of diluent:

volume of diluent = final volume − initial volume

volume of diluent = 750 mL − 300 mL = 450 mL

Hint: In the dilution equation, the abbreviations are as follows:

- C1 is the initial concentration.
- Q1 is the initial quantity.
- C2 is the final concentration.
- Q2 is the final quantity.

The initial concentration will always be larger than the final concentration and the initial volume will always be smaller than the final volume. This is because in order to break down the concentration, a diluent needs to be added, which results in a larger volume and a smaller concentration.

(409)

A pharmacy technician is asked to dilute 300 g of a 20% lidocaine solution to a 10% concentration. How much is the final quantity of lidocaine?

A. 600 mg
B. 150 g
C. 700 mg
D. 600 g

(410)

If 450 mL of a 20 mg/mL solution was diluted to 5 mg/mL, what would be the final volume?

A. 0.2 mL
B. 113 mL
C. 1,800 mL
D. 800 mL

(411)

D. 600 g

Rationale:

Use the dilution equation:

$(C1)(Q1) = (C2)(Q2)$

$20\% \times (300\ g) = 10\% \times (x)$

$x = (20 \times 300)/10 = 600\ g$

(410)

C. 1,800 mL

Rationale:

Use the dilution equation:

$(C1)(Q1) = (C2)(Q2)$

$(20\ mg/mL)(450\ mL) = (5\ mg/mL)(x); x = (20 \times 450)/(5) = 1,800\ mL$

Hint: Remember final concentration is always greater than the initial concentration.

If the initial concentration was given in different units than the final concentration or vice versa, you need to convert to the same denomination before using the dilution equation.

(411)

How many 300 mg tablets are needed to make 1,500 mL of a 1:400 solution?

A. 12 tablets
B. 13 tablets
C. 1 tablet
D. 20 tablets

(412)

After diluting 8 kg of 30% hydrocortisone ointment to 2.5% strength, how many 28 g tubes can be filled?

A. 3,428 tubes
B. 667 tubes
C. 96 tubes
D. 336 tubes

(413)

B. 13 tablets

Rationale:

Step 1: Calculate the amount needed in milligrams:

1:400 = 1 g/400 mL

1 g/400 mL = x /1,500 mL

$x = (1 \times 1,500)/400 = 3.75$ g = 3,750 mg

Step 2: Figure out how many tablets are needed:

quantity to be dispensed = desired dose ÷ dose available

3,750 mg ÷ 300 mg = 12.5 or 13 tablets

(412)

A. 3,428 tubes

Rationale:

Step 1: Convert the following:

8 kg = 8,000 gm

Step 2: Calculate the final quantity using the dilution equation:

(C1) × (Q1) = (C2) × (Q2)

(30%) (8,000 g) = (2.5%) (x)

$x = (30 \times 8,000)/2.5 = 96,000$ g

Step 3: Calculate the quantity of tubes that can be filled:

96,000 g ÷ 28 g = 3,428 tubes

(413)

What is 1:125 in percent strength?

A. 125%
B. 0.8%
C. 0.008%
D. 0.08%

(414)

How many omeprazole 20 mg capsules would be required to make the following omeprazole solution?

Omeprazole 2%

Sodium bicarbonate 50%

Qs with 0.45% normal saline to 50 mL

A. 4 capsules
B. 50 capsules
C. 125 capsules
D. 200 capsules

(415)

B. 0.8%

Rationale:

1:125 = 1/125 when written as a fraction

Convert to percent strength by dividing the numerator by the denominator and multiplying by 100:

(1/125) × 100 = 0.8%

Or you can write this as a proportion:

1/125 = x/100

x = (1 × 125)/100 = 0.8%

(414)

B. 50 capsules

Rationale:

Step 1: Calculate quantity of omeprazole needed to make a 50 mL solution:

2/100 = x/50

x = (2 × 50)/100 = 1 g

Step 2: Calculate the quantity of omeprazole capsules needed:

1 g = 1,000 mg

1,000 ÷ 20 = 50 capsules

(415)

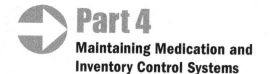

The pharmacy filing systems include all of the following EXCEPT:

A. a folder for all medications including Schedules II–V

B. a folder for Schedule II, a folder for Schedules III–V stamped with a red C in the lower right-hand corner, and a folder for all other prescriptions

C. a folder for Schedules II–V with Schedule III–V prescriptions stamped with a red C in the lower right-hand corner, and a folder for all other prescriptions

D. a folder for Schedule II, a folder for Schedules III–V and all other prescriptions, with Schedules III–V being identified with a red C stamp in the lower right-hand corner

(416)

A. a folder for all medications including Schedules II–V

Rationale:

There are three filing methods: One is a three-folder system and two are two-folder systems. They are ordered as follows:

	Filing System # 1	Filing System # 2	Filing System # 3
Folder 1	Schedule II prescriptions	Schedule II prescriptions	Schedule II prescriptions and Schedule III, IV, V (III to V prescriptions need to be marked with a red "C" at the lower right-hand corner for easy identification)
Folder 2	Schedules III, IV, V	Schedules III, IV, V, and all other prescriptions (III to V prescriptions need to be marked with a red "C" at the lower right-hand corner for easy identification)	All other prescriptions
Folder 3	All other prescriptions		

(416)

If a pharmacy has an annual purchasing cost of $2,400,000 and the average cost of the inventory on hand is $140,000, what is the turnover rate?

A. 15
B. 16
C. 17
D. 18

(417)

If a pharmacy has an annual purchasing cost of $1,400,000 and the inventory cost at the beginning of a particular month was $200,000 and $400,000 at the end of the month, what is the turnover rate?

A. 4
B. 5
C. 6
D. 7

(418)

C. 17

Rationale:

Use the following formula:

inventory turnover rate = cost of annual purchases ÷ value of average inventory on hand

$2,400,000 ÷ $140,000 = 17 turns

Since the turnover in this case is high, the pharmacy can fix that by ordering more stock to last a longer time.

(417)

B. 5

Rationale:

Step 1: Calculate the average inventory:

Average inventory = (beginning inventory + ending inventory)/2

(200,000 + 400,000) ÷ 2 = $300,000

Step 2: Calculate the inventory turnover rate using the following formula:

inventory turnover rate = cost of annual purchases ÷ value of average inventory on hand

$1,400,000 ÷ $300,000 = 4.6 or 5 turns

(418)

A pharmacy has a minimum/maximum inventory level of 20/40 for hydroxyzine 25 mg tablets. If 15 tablets were left in stock, what is the minimum amount of tablets that should be reordered?

A. 20 tablets
B. 40 tablets
C. 25 tablets
D. 10 tablets

(419)

Expired or unused medications can be returned to which of the following facilities?

A. centralized warehouse
B. manufacturer
C. wholesaler
D. all of the above can accept returns

(420)

C. 25 tablets

Rationale:

40 − 15 = 25 tablets

Hint: The reordering quantity should bring the periodic automatic replenishment (PAR) level up to the maximum quantity required. So, the amount to be reordered is always the maximum quantity minus the amount on hand.

(419)

D. all of the above can accept returns

Rationale:

Medications are pulled from stock 3 to 4 months before they expire and returned to a centralized warehouse, manufacturer, or the wholesaler for partial credit. Medications with open seals or that are partially used cannot be returned and have to be discarded in a biohazard container.

(420)

According to the Controlled Substances Act, which of the following statements is true regarding disposal of unused or expired controlled medications?

A. They may be returned to the manufacturer.
B. They may be flushed down the drain.
C. They may be returned to reverse distributors.
D. all of the above

(421)

Which of the following medications is listed as hazardous waste?

A. furosemide
B. metoprolol
C. some chemotherapy agents
D. all of the above

(422)

D. all of the above

Rationale:

According to the controlled substances act, the following is true regarding disposal of unused or expired controlled medications:

- They may be returned to the manufacturer.

- They may be destroyed and documented following state guidelines. This includes medication flushing down the drain.

- They may be returned to reverse distributors or automated return companies.

(421)

C. some chemotherapy agents

Rationale:

Nitroglycerin, warfarin, and some chemotherapy agents are considered hazardous waste. Others include: arsenic trioxide, epinephrine, nicotine, physostigmine, physostigmine salicylate, chlorambucil, cyclophosphamide, daunomycin, melphalan, mitomycin C, streptozotocin, and uracil mustard.

(422)

**Where should hazardous pharmaceutical waste
be disposed?**

A. municipal waste landfills
B. hazardous waste disposal facilities
C. municipal incinerators
D. medical waste plants

(423)

**Which of the following organizations governs the
management of pharmaceutical hazardous waste?**

A. FDA
B. DEA
C. EPA
D. TJC

(424)

B. hazardous waste disposal facilities

Rationale:

Hazardous pharmaceutical waste must be disposed of in approved hazardous waste containers to be transported by a hazardous waste transporter to hazardous waste disposal facilities.

(423)

C. EPA

Rationale:

- The Environmental Protection Agency (EPA) governs the management of pharmaceutical hazardous waste.

- The FDA is the Food and Drug Administration, which regulates prescription and over-the-counter drugs.

- The DEA is the Drug Enforcement Agency, which deals with controlled substances.

- The TJC is The Joint Commission, which accredits healthcare organizations.

(424)

Which of the following tablets cannot be crushed?

A. Ecotrin 325 mg
B. aspirin 325 mg
C. furosemide 20 mg
D. glyburide 2.5 mg

(425)

How are pharmaceutical labels disposed of in a long-term care facility?

A. regular trash
B. hazardous waste container
C. confidential data shredding bucket
D. biohazard waste container

(426)

A. Ecotrin 325 mg

Rationale:

Ecotrin is enteric coated aspirin. The enteric coating protects the aspirin against stomach acid to be dissolved in the enteric or small intestine. Crushing the tablet would interfere with its formulation and make it ineffective. Other drugs with special formulations such as extended-release or long-acting drugs also should not be crushed.

(425)

C. confidential data shredding bucket

Rationale:

To comply with HIPAA regulations, long-term care facilities shred all pharmaceutical labels that contain private information or personal identifiers. Confidential data should be disposed of in a confidential data shredding bucket for later destruction. They should never be discarded in a regular trash container unless any private information is erased or properly concealed.

(426)

Where should the gowns and gloves used in chemotherapy compounding be disposed?

A. regular trash
B. sharps container
C. yellow chemo waste bag
D. red biohazard bag

(427)

Where should partially used chemotherapy vials be disposed?

A. regular trash
B. biohazard waste container
C. yellow chemo waste bag
D. yellow chemotherapy waste sharps container

(428)

C. yellow chemo waste bag

Rationale:

All protective equipment used to make or administer chemo medication is considered hazardous waste and must be disposed of in a yellow chemo waste bag because of possible contamination. Sharps containers can be used for discarding non-chemo vials and non-chemo syringes and needles. Red biohazard bags are used for disposal of blood-contaminated material or other potentially infectious material.

(427)

D. yellow chemotherapy waste sharps container

Rationale:

All chemotherapy vials, syringes, needles, and empty IV bags should be disposed of in a yellow chemotherapy waste sharps container so they may be incinerated or autoclaved because they are considered dangerous. Other waste such as gowns, gloves, goggles, tubing, and wipes should be disposed of in a yellow chemotherapy bag. The biohazard waste container is reserved for needles, vials, syringes, and chemical waste that is noncytotoxic.

(428)

Which of the following insurance plans would cover citizens with end-stage renal disease?

A. TRICARE
B. CHAMPVA
C. Medicare
D. Medicaid

(429)

C. Medicare

Rationale:

TRICARE, CHAMPVA, Medicare, and Medicaid are all government programs. However:

- TRICARE covers military personnel on active duty, retired military personnel, and their dependents.

- CHAMPVA covers veterans with permanent disabilities related to service and their dependents.

- Medicare is federally funded and covers citizens 65 years of age or older, people with disabilities, spouses of entitled individuals, and people with end-stage renal disease.

- Medicaid is funded by federal and state government. It covers individuals with low income who cannot afford medical care.

(429)

What is the name of the government agency that administers Medicare and Medicaid services?

A. CMS
B. DEA
C. FDA
D. TJC

(430)

The Medicare prescription drug improvement and modernization act (MMA) of 2003 led to the development of which part of Medicare?

A. Medicare Part A
B. Medicare Part B
C. Medicare Part C
D. Medicare Part D

(431)

A. CMS

Rationale:

- The Centers for Medicare and Medicaid Services (CMS) is a U.S. federal government agency that administers all laws and policies related to Medicare and Medicaid.

- DEA is the Drug Enforcement Agency, which deals with regulations related to narcotics.

- FDA is the Food and Drug Administration, which deals with regulations pertaining to all prescription drugs and over-the-counter medications.

- TJC is The Joint Commission, formerly known as The Joint Commission on Accreditation of Healthcare Organizations (JCAHO). This organization accredits healthcare institutions.

(430)

D. Medicare part D

Rationale:

- Medicare Part A deals with inpatient services such as hospital stays, care in skilled nursing facilities, hospice care, and home health care.

- Medicare Part B covers outpatient visits.

- Medicare Part C combines coverage for parts A and B.

- Medicare Part D is a voluntary insurance benefit for outpatient prescription coverage enacted as part of the Drug Improvement and Modernization Act (MMA) of 2003.

(431)

**Which of the following is a system that automatically
deducts scanned items from the inventory, making it easy to
reorder and keep track of medication counts?**

A. set order points
B. perpetual inventory
C. point of sale (POS)
D. turnover rate

(432)

C. point of sale (POS)

Rationale:

- The set order points system is based on minimum and maximum ordering points. This requires visual inspection of stocks to determine the reordering quantity for each item available in the pharmacy. If the information is processed through the computer, it will make it easier to determine the needed inventory levels.

- The perpetual inventory system utilizes a computer system to scan all new items received by the pharmacy. All items sold or dispensed are automatically deducted from the inventory. This system can also keep track of minimum and maximum levels if they are inputted into the computer. However, this requires periodic verification of stock against computer data.

- The point-of-sale (POS) system utilizes a computer to keep a perpetual inventory. All items sold are scanned and automatically deducted from the inventory. This makes it easy to reorder and keep track of medication counts.

- The turnover rate determines how frequently during a particular year new stock is purchased to replenish the inventory.

(432)

Which of the following statements is true regarding why
pharmacies prefer purchasing most of their stock from
wholesalers or distributors?

A. It is difficult to deal with all the different manufacturers.
B. Manufacturers stock most medications at competitive prices.
C. Manufacturers make daily deliveries and provide systems for
   ordering medications.
D. all of the above

(433)

According to the DEA, how often must a full inventory of
controlled substances take place?

A. every 3 years
B. every day
C. every 2 years
D. twice per year

(434)

A. It is difficult to deal with all the different manufacturers.

Rationale:

Pharmacies prefer purchasing most of their stock from wholesalers or distributors because:

- It is difficult to deal with all the different manufacturers.

- Wholesalers stock most medications at competitive prices.

- Wholesalers make daily deliveries and provide systems for ordering medications.

Pharmacies purchase from manufacturers' special orders and backordered items.

(433)

C. every 2 years

Rationale:

In accordance with DEA rules, every person should maintain an inventory of controlled substances in stock when they first engage in dispensing these medications and a new inventory should be taken every 2 years thereafter.

(434)

Where should Schedule II narcotics be stored?

A. separately in a secure place
B. dispersed on the shelf with other prescription medications
C. stored next to oral chemotherapy medications
D. in the same compartment as investigational drugs

(435)

How soon should the supplier be paid for stock purchases?

A. as soon as the order is placed
B. as soon as the order is delivered
C. within 30 days from the date of delivery
D. within 1 year from the date of purchase

(436)

New stock items should be inspected for which of the following?

A. expiration date
B. damage during shipping
C. item names and quantities
D. all of the above

(437)

A. separately in a secure place

Rationale:

Schedule II narcotics should be stored separately in a secure place, preferably in a locked compartment because they are highly abused. They should not be dispersed on the shelf with other prescription medication.

Chemotherapy medications and investigational drugs should also be stored separate from all other medications.

(435)

C. within 30 days from the date of delivery

Rationale:

The supplier must be paid for stock purchases within 30 days from the date of delivery. Otherwise, service charges may be added to the unpaid balance, which will result in higher costs.

(436)

D. all of the above

Rationale:

All newly received stock items should be inspected for item names and quantities, expiration dates, and any damage during shipping. Damaged and expired or soon-to-be-expired stock received can be returned to the wholesaler for credit.

(437)

Which of the following items can be returned to reverse distributors or the manufacturer for credit?

A. partially used medication vials
B. partially used ointments
C. expired drugs
D. reconstituted suspensions

(438)

What is the proper way of handling an unopened prescription vial that was returned by the patient?

A. credit the patient and return the medication to stock
B. the medication should be credited and destroyed within 72 hours
C. a destruction record should be kept on file
D. both B and C

(439)

C. expired drugs

Rationale:

Reverse distributors sort through unused or expired medications. Partially used or reconstituted medications are considered waste and cannot be returned for credit.

(438)

D. both B and C

Rationale:

Returned medications that are not sealed and intact cannot be returned to stock. It is difficult to determine if medications within a prescription vial were adulterated, mishandled, or somehow contaminated. It is safer to discard them than to reuse them.

Returned medications that are unexpired—in an original sealed container, and with unaltered packaging and labels—can be returned to stock if deemed appropriate by the pharmacist.

(439)

Which of the following statements is NOT true regarding
reverse distributors or automated return companies?

A. Reverse distributors sort through unused or expired medications
to determine which can be returned to the manufacturer or
wholesaler for credit.
B. Reverse distributors warehouses have to be licensed by the
Department of Health, Bureau of Statewide Pharmaceutical
Services.
C. Partial intravenous medications, partially used vials, and
partially used ointments or creams can be returned to reverse
distributors for credit.
D. Reverse distributors accept the return of recalled items.

(440)

Which of the following statements is true regarding generic
drugs?

A. Drugs have many brand names but only one generic name.
B. Generic drugs are less effective than brand names.
C. Generic drugs are just as expensive as brand names.
D. Insurances would cover brand name drugs if the patient does not
want the generic alternative.

(441)

C. Partial intravenous medications, partially used vials, and partially used ointments or creams can be returned to reverse distributors for credit.

Rationale:

- Reverse distributors sort through unused or expired medications to determine which can be returned to the manufacturer or wholesaler for credit.

- Reverse distributors warehouses have to be licensed by the state Department of Health, Bureau of Statewide Pharmaceutical Services.

- Reverse distributors accept the return of recalled items.

- Partial intravenous medications, partially used vials, and partially used ointments or creams cannot be returned to reverse distributors for credit.

(440)

A. Drugs have many brand names but only one generic name.

Rationale:

- Drugs have many brand names but only one generic name.

- Generic drugs are just as effective as brand names.

- Generic drugs are less expensive than brand names.

- Insurances would cover a brand name drug only if the doctor states that it is medically necessary. Otherwise, the patient would have to pay the difference in cost.

(441)

Which of the following is an example of quality assurance
and validation testing performed by pharmacy technicians
who compound sterile products?

A. media refill test procedure
B. media fill test procedure
C. glove fingertip sampling procedure
D. both B and C

(442)

Which of the following *Orange Book* equivalency ratings
indicates that a generic drug is not bioequivalent to its
respective brand name?

A. AB
B. BP
C. AO
D. AT

(443)

Which of the following is NOT a true statement regarding
closed formularies?

A. A physician needs permission to order any medication not
   included on the formulary.
B. Less expensive medications are stocked for cost saving reasons.
C. They allow physicians to order any medication.
D. The list of approved medications is limited.

(444)

D. both B and C

Rationale:

The media fill test and the glove fingertip sampling procedures are examples of quality assurance and validation testing performed by pharmacy technicians who compound sterile products.

(442)

B. BP

Rationale:

Any rating that starts with an "A" indicates that the drug is bioequivalent. However, drug ratings that start with a "B" indicate that the drug is not bioequivalent.

(443)

C. They allow physicians to order any medication.

Rationale:

The following statements are true regarding closed formularies:

- Closed formularies require physicians to ask for permission for ordering medications not included on the formulary.

- Less expensive medications are stocked for cost saving reasons.

- The list of approved medications is limited.

- Open formularies allow physicians to order any medication.

(444)

Which of the following refers to the process of moving
products with an early expiration date to the front of a shelf
and placing products with later expiration dates in the back?

A. stock rotation
B. stock depletion
C. stock turn
D. stock arrangement

(445)

Which of the following are NOT crash or code cart
medications?

A. amiodarone injection
B. epinephrine Abboject
C. sumatriptan injection
D. atropine Abboject

(446)

Which of the following statements is true regarding beyond-
use dating of repackaged medications?

A. The expiration date should be 6 months or 25% of the remaining
   manufacturer's expiration, whichever comes first.
B. It should be 1 year after the manufacturer's expiration date.
C. It should be 1 year from the date of repackaging without regard
   to the manufacturer's expiration date.
D. The expiration date of repackaged medications should be the
   same as the one provided by the manufacturer.

(447)

A. stock rotation

Rationale:

Stock rotation is the process of moving products with an early expiration date to the front of a shelf and placing products with later expiration dates in the back so that stock with an earlier expiration date can be used first. This reduces medication waste and therefore is also a cost-saving strategy.

(445)

C. sumatriptan injection

Rationale:

Code cart medications are emergency medications used to rescue individuals in or near a coding situation. They are usually injectable medications used in cardiac resuscitation. Sumatriptan is a migraine prophylactic medication.

(446)

A. The expiration date should be 6 months or 25% of the remaining manufacturer's expiration, whichever comes first.

Rationale:

The general rule for beyond-use dating of repackaged medications is that it should be 6 months or 25% of the remaining manufacturer's expiration, whichever comes first, unless otherwise indicated by the manufacturer.

(447)

How soon before the expiration date should medications be pulled off the shelf?

A. 1 week
B. 1 month
C. 2 months
D. 3 months

(448)

Which of the following would not be an adequate reason for recalling medications?

A. contamination
B. mislabeling or mispackaging
C. good manufacturing
D. all of the above

(449)

D. 3 months

Rationale:

Medications about to expire should be pulled off the shelf 3 to
4 months ahead of the expiration date. This is a practice done by
pharmacies to ensure that available medications are not expired or
deteriorated.

(448)

C. good manufacturing

Rationale:

Contamination, mislabeling or mispackaging, and poor
manufacturing are all adequate reasons for recalling medications.
Recalls can range from severe to non-life threatening as follows:

- Class 1 recall: There is a high probability that the use of the
  medication will cause severe adverse health consequence
  or death.

- Class 2 recall: The use of the medication will cause a
  temporary or reversible adverse health consequence.

- Class 3 recall: The use of the medication is not likely to cause
  any adverse health consequences.

(449)

Which of the following medications should not be crushed?

A. olanzapine 10 mg tablet
B. Cardizem LA 300 mg tablet
C. pravastatin 20 mg tablet
D. lisinopril 10 mg tablet

(450)

B. Cardizem LA 300 mg tablet

Rationale:

All medications with extended-release formulation should not be crushed. Other medications that should not be crushed are identified by the following abbreviations:

- CD = controlled delivery
- CR = controlled release
- DA = delayed absorption
- DR = delayed release
- EC = enteric coated
- ER = enteric release
- GC = granules within capsule
- HGC = hard gelatin capsule
- IR = irritant
- LA = long acting
- LC = liquid within a capsule
- LF = liquid filled
- MMI = mucous membrane irritant
- PC = protective coating
- SL = sublingual
- SPT = strong, persistent taste
- SR = slow release
- SSR = sustained release
- TR = timed release
- TS = taste
- XL = extended release
- XR = extended release

(450)

Who can sign the record to validate for narcotic delivery to
automated dispensing systems within a hospital?

A. LPN
B. RN
C. pharmacist
D. pharmacy technician

(451)

Another name for a single supplier that provides pharmacies
with a major portion of the system's purchases at lower
cost is:

A. prime supplier
B. manufacturer
C. group purchasing organization
D. sole provider

(452)

B. RN

Rationale:

Only a registered nurse (RN) can sign to verify delivery of narcotics. Accounting for narcotics is not in the LPN's scope of practice.

(451)

A. prime supplier

Rationale:

Prime supplier or vendor is another name for the single supplier that provides pharmacies with a major portion of the system's purchases at lower cost. Pharmacies tend to have a contract for purchasing supplies from a prime supplier that would provide them with most of the medications they need at competitive prices.

(452)

Which of the following organizations regulates medical devices?

A. DEA
B. CMS
C. FDA
D. TJC

(453)

Which of the following is the newest method of inventory control used in management of set order points?

A. purchase order
B. want book
C. handheld device
D. none of the above

(454)

C. FDA

Rationale:

- The DEA is the Drug Enforcement Agency, which deals with regulations related to narcotics.

- The Centers for Medicare and Medicaid Services (CMS) is a U.S. federal government agency that administers all laws and policies related to Medicare and Medicaid.

- The FDA is the Food and Drug Administration, which regulates medical devices and deals with regulations pertaining to all prescription drugs and over-the-counter medications.

- The TJC is The Joint Commission, formerly known as The Joint Commission on Accreditation of Healthcare Organizations (JCAHO). This organization accredits healthcare institutions.

(453)

C. handheld device

Rationale:

Want book is an old and widely used method of inventory control used in management of set order points. This method is now replaced by the wireless handheld device, which can look up items by barcode scan and allow for the information to be directly transferred to the main computer ordering system.

(454)

Total control of quality of drugs is the responsibility of:

A. the pharmacy director
B. all pharmacy staff
C. the nursing supervisor
D. all of the above

(455)

**Quality control of medications encompasses which
of the following?**

A. formulation, compounding, and dispensing
B. packaging, purchasing, and storage
C. distribution of medication to the patient
D. all of the above

(456)

B. all pharmacy staff

Rationale:

Quality control of drugs is the responsibility of the entire pharmacy department, which includes the pharmacy director, the pharmacists, and the pharmacy technicians. This guarantees the dispensing of the right medication to the right patient at the right time and prevents medication errors.

(455)

D. all of the above

Rationale:

Quality control of medication encompasses all of the following:

- Formulation, compounding, and dispensing
- Packaging, purchasing, and storage
- Distribution of medication to the patient

Failure to properly complete one of the above steps can lead to a preventable medication error.

(456)

Which of the following negotiates medication prices for institutions but does not make the actual purchases?

A. drug manufacturer
B. wholesaler
C. group purchasing organization
D. government

(457)

Which of the following drugs can crystallize at very low temperatures?

A. nitroglycerin
B. amiodarone
C. mannitol
D. sodium bicarbonate

(458)

How long is nitroglycerin sublingual stable after opening the container?

A. 30 days
B. 6 months
C. 12 months
D. 1 year

(459)

C. group purchasing organization

Rationale:

The group purchasing organization negotiates medication prices for institutions but does not make the actual purchases. These organizations assist in promoting quality healthcare and in effectively managing expenses.

(457)

C. mannitol

Rationale:

Mannitol should be stored at room temperature. If it crystallizes, it should be placed in an autoclave for at least 20 minutes until all crystals have dissolved. The vials should not be used if crystals are present.

(458)

B. 6 months

Rationale:

Nitroglycerin sublingual is only stable for 6 months after opening the container. The medication will not be effective if it loses its potency.

(459)

Which of the following represents drug diversion cases?

A. the use of addictive drugs for nontherapeutic purposes
B. the illegal distribution of drugs
C. prescription forgery
D. all of the above

(460)

As long as the manufacturer's storage requirements are met, what is the beyond-use date of a multidose vial such as insulin injection after opening?

A. 1 week
B. 14 days
C. 28 days
D. 30 days

(461)

Which of the following accurately defines sterility of compounded sterile products (CSPs)?

A. lack of color change
B. no precipitates
C. free of microorganisms
D. both A and B

(462)

D. all of the above

Rationale:

The following are examples of drug diversion:

- The use of addictive drugs for nontherapeutic purposes
- The illegal distribution of drugs
- Prescription forgery such as faking prescriptions to obtain medications illegally

(460)

C. 28 days

Rationale:

Multidose vials are stable for 28 days unless otherwise specified by the manufacturer and as long as the manufacturer storage requirements are met. For instance, insulin is stable for 28 days at room temperature and until the manufacturer's expiration date if kept refrigerated.

(461)

C. free of microorganisms

Rationale:

A sterile CSP is free of microorganisms. This is important because nonsterile products given intravenously could lead to a systemic infection, which would be hazardous to health.

(462)

Which of the following can result from lack of stability
of a CSP?

A. color change
B. precipitate formation
C. chemical degradation
D. all of the above

(463)

Where should Xalatan eye drops be stored?

A. on the shelf at room temperature
B. in the refrigerator
C. in the freezer
D. in a warmer

(464)

Which of the following medications should not be protected
from light?

A. nitroglycerin
B. nitrofurantoin
C. methylprednisolone
D. all of the above

(465)

D. all of the above

Rationale:

Lack of stability results in chemical and physical characteristic
changes such as color change, precipitate formation, and chemical
degradation. Once a CSP loses the original chemical and physical
characteristic, it should be discarded to avoid severe health
consequences.

(463)

B. in the refrigerator

Rationale:

Xalatan eye drops or latanoprost should be refrigerated per
the manufacturer's recommendation. At room temperature, the
medication loses its stability.

(464)

B. nitrofurantoin

Rationale:

Nitroglycerin, sulfadiazine, and methylprednisolone should all be
protected from light because otherwise they would deteriorate and
lose potency. Nitrofurantoin is not light sensitive. However, most
medications should be protected from light.

(465)

Which of the following is not true regarding just-in-time ordering?

A. supplies items close to the time of use
B. reduces large inventories
C. increases cost and space requirements
D. all of the above

(466)

Which of the following insurances requires higher copayments but allows patients a wide range of access to out-of-network physicians?

A. HMO
B. PPO
C. Medicare
D. TRICARE

(467)

C. increases cost and space requirements

Rationale:

Just-in-time ordering supplies items close to the time of use, reduces large inventories, and decreases cost and space requirements.

(466)

B. PPO

Rationale:

- The preferred provider organization (PPO) requires higher copayments but allows patients a wide range of access to out-of-network physicians.

- The health maintenance organization (HMO) requires lower copayments but gives patients restricted access to out-of-network physicians.

- Medicare is federally funded and covers citizens 65 years of age or older, people with disabilities, spouses of entitled individuals, and people with end-stage renal disease.

- TRICARE covers military personnel on active duty, retired military personnel, and dependents of military personnel.

(467)

How long are drug patents effective?

A. 20 years from the date of patent application filing
B. 20 years from the time the drug is placed on the market
C. 20 years after the end of phase II trials
D. 20 years after the end of phase III trials

(468)

Which clinical trial phase involves studies done on 1,000 to 5,000 patient volunteers to confirm effectiveness and monitor adverse effects associated with long-term use of an experimental drug?

A. phase I
B. phase II
C. phase III
D. phase IV

(469)

How long should records for controlled substances be stored?

A. 30 days
B. 1 year
C. 2 years
D. 7 years

(470)

A. 20 years from the date of patent application filing

Rationale:

A drug patent is effective for 20 years from the date of patent application filing. After a drug patent runs out, competitor manufacturer industries are allowed to produce generics of the drug.

(468)

C. phase III

Rationale:

- Phase I involves 20 to 100 patient volunteers and is intended to determine safety and dosage of an experimental drug.
- Phase II involves 100 to 500 patient volunteers and is intended to evaluate effectiveness and look for side effects of an experimental drug.
- Phase III involves 1,000 to 5,000 patient volunteers to confirm effectiveness and monitor adverse effects associated with long-term use of an experimental drug.
- Phase IV involves postmarketing studies required by the FDA to determine long-term safety of an experimental drug.

(469)

C. 2 years

Rationale:

According to the DEA, all controlled substances records should be stored for a minimum of 2 years to provide accountability of all controlled substances received and dispensed in case of errors.

(470)

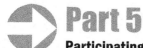

Part 5

Participating in the Administration and Management of Pharmacy Practice

---

If a nurse calls with a question regarding compatibility of two different medications, a pharmacy technician receiving the call should:

A. answer the question to the best of his or her knowledge
B. forward the call to the pharmacist
C. ask another pharmacy technician for help
D. place the nurse on hold, look up the answer in one of the pharmacy reference books, and then provide the best answer

(471)

What is another name for a decentralized pharmacy unit?

A. remote
B. satellite
C. internal
D. external

(472)

B. forward the call to the pharmacist

Rationale:

Drug compatibility questions and all other medication questions should be directed to the pharmacist's attention.

(471)

B. satellite

Rationale:

A decentralized pharmacy unit is also known as a *satellite unit*. In large hospitals, the main inpatient pharmacy is also known as the *central pharmacy*. Smaller satellite pharmacies exist in different departments (i.e., operating room pharmacy, intensive care unit pharmacy, emergency department pharmacy, etc.). This improves medication delivery time, which is important for providing quality care. Satellite pharmacies are stocked by the central pharmacy.

(472)

Which of the following commonly accounts for insurance claim rejection?

A. invalid date of birth
B. loss of insurance coverage
C. maximum benefit has been reached
D. all of the above

(473)

How often is the temperature of controlled-temperature areas of a pharmacy recorded?

A. daily
B. weekly
C. monthly
D. twice every year

(474)

D. all of the above

Rationale:

Any of the following may lead to insurances rejecting claims:

- Invalid patient information; this includes error typing name, heath plan number, insurance card number, date of birth, or relationship to the cardholder

- Patient loss of insurance coverage

- Maximum benefit has been reached

- Early refill request

- Selected drug is not covered

(473)

A. daily

Rationale:

It is important to maintain daily temperature logs of controlled-temperature areas of pharmacy to make sure that medications are stored at the appropriate temperatures and they are not deteriorating. Any fluctuation in temperature due to malfunctioning of equipment may lead to medication spoilage.

(474)

Which of the following organizations enforces health
and safety in the workplace?

A. OSHA
B. FDA
C. DEA
D. TJC

(475)

How many continuing education credits are required
over the course of 2 years by a certified pharmacy
technician?

A. 10
B. 20
C. 30
D. 40

(476)

A. OSHA

Rationale:

- OSHA is the Occupational Safety and Health Administration, which enforces health and safety in the workplace.

- The FDA is the Food and Drug Administration, which regulates prescription and over-the-counter drugs.

- The DEA is the Drug Enforcement Agency, which deals with controlled substances.

- The TJC is The Joint Commission, which accredits healthcare organizations.

(475)

B. 20

Rationale:

A certified pharmacy technician is required to complete 20 continuing education (CEs) credits over the course of 2 years or 10 CEs per year. At least 1 of the 20 CEs should be in pharmacy law.

(476)

What is the meaning of the abbreviation USP?

A. unique selling proposition
B. United States pharmacist
C. United States Pharmacopeia
D. uniform stability of pharmaceuticals

(477)

Why should nursing units be inspected or inventoried?

A. to remove deteriorated or expired medications
B. to ensure overall cleanliness and organization of the medication
   storage area
C. to ensure proper temperature of refrigerators containing
   medications and that no foods, beverages, or culture media are
   stored with medications
D. all of the above

(478)

C. United States Pharmacopeia

Rationale:

The United States Pharmacopeia is a nongovernmental organization that sets standards for medications, food ingredients, and dietary supplements to be followed by manufacturers and regulatory agencies. The standards are intended to ensure strength, quality, purity, and consistency of these various products.

(477)

D. all of the above

Rationale:

Nursing units are inspected for the following reasons:

- To remove deteriorated or expired medications
- To ensure overall cleanliness and organization of medication storage area
- To ensure proper temperature of refrigerators containing medications and that no foods, beverages, or culture media are stored with medications

Nursing units are inspected by pharmacy staff once every month.

(478)

Which of the following is an equipment required by law to be available in every pharmacy?

A. digital balance
B. class A balance
C. spatula
D. pill counting tray

(479)

The cost of metoprolol tablets is $200 per 50 tablets. How much will the cost be for a prescription of 60 tablets if the patient is eligible for a 20% senior citizen discount?

A. $240
B. $220
C. $192
D. $48

(480)

B. class A balance

Rationale:

A class A balance or torsion balance is required by law to be available in every pharmacy. This balance has a sensitivity requirement of 6 mg and can accurately weigh a minimum of 120 mg up to 15 g.

(479)

C. $192

Rationale:

Step 1: Calculate the cost of 60 tablets using ratio proportion:

$200/50 tablets $= x/60$ tablets

$x = (200 \times 60)/50 = \$240$

Step 2: Calculate the cost of the tablets after discount:

$$20\% = \frac{20}{100}$$

$$= \frac{20}{100} \times (240) = \$48 \text{ discount}$$
Cost after discount $= \$240 - \$48 = \$192$

(480)

How often should the laminar airflow hood (LAH) be certified?

A. once every 2 years
B. every 6 months
C. three times per year
D. every 4 months

(481)

Which of the following can be transported via a pneumatic tube?

A. rituximab
B. atenolol 50 mg tablets
C. Epogen
D. all of the above

(482)

Which of the following is necessary to have while transporting chemotherapy medications?

A. a phone
B. a pager
C. a spill kit
D. a respirator

(483)

B. every 6 months

Rationale:

The LAH should be certified every 6 months and whenever the hood is moved by an independent certification agency. Certification is done to ensure operational efficiency and efficacy.

(481)

B. atenolol 50 mg tablets

Rationale:

Medications that cannot be transported via pneumatic tube include hazardous medications, controlled substances, and medications in glass containers.

(482)

C. a spill kit

Rationale:

A spill kit is necessary to have while transporting chemotherapy medications. A spill kit contains: goggles, gown, latex-free gloves, show covers, respirator mask, scoop and brush, absorbent towels, hazardous drug exposure form, and spill control pillows. These items can be used for the cleanup and containment of an accidental chemotherapy spill.

(483)

Which of the following filters removes particulate matter and bacteria that may have been introduced during the preparation of an epidural?

A. 0.22 micron
B. 5 micron
C. 10 micron
D. 15 micron

(484)

Which of the following can help reduce medication errors?

A. knowing the common look-alike and sound-alike medications
B. keeping hazardous medications in a separate storage area
C. always questioning bad handwriting
D. all of the above

(485)

A. 0.22 micron

Rationale:

A 0.22 micron filter is used to remove particulate matter and bacteria that may have been introduced during the preparation of an epidural. A 5 micron filter is used to filter out glass particles when preparing sterile products from ampoules.

(484)

D. all of the above

Rationale:

Knowing the common look-alike and sound-alike medications, keeping hazardous medications in a separate storage area, and always questioning bad handwriting are all good medication error-reduction strategies. Other error-reduction strategies include: using the Tall Man lettering system, avoiding the use of abbreviations, checking medication names on bottles against the labels and the original order, and asking questions when in doubt.

(485)

A pharmacy technician misinterpreted a prescription that read: "insulin 10u" for 100 units of insulin. What type of error has occurred?

A. assumption error
B. selection error
C. capture error
D. extra dose error

(486)

According to USP 797, how often should a compounder performing low- to medium-risk preparations undergo validation testing?

A. every month
B. every 6 months
C. every year
D. every 2 years

(487)

A. assumption error

Rationale:

- An assumption error occurs when information that cannot be interpreted is guessed.

- A selection error occurs when the wrong drug is selected.

- A capture error is created when an individual's attention is diverted, causing an error to be made.

- An extra dose error occurs when more doses than were prescribed are dispensed.

(486)

C. every year

Rationale:

A compounder performing low- to medium-risk preparations should undergo validation testing once every year per USP 797. The media-fill test or glove fingertip sampling ensures the competency of the compounding technician.

(487)

According to USP 797, how often should a compounder
performing high-risk preparations undergo validation
testing?

A. every month
B. every 6 months
C. every year
D. every 2 years

(488)

Which of the following is the most effective way to prevent
contamination and the spread of infection within a hospital?

A. taking vitamin C
B. wearing a face mask
C. hand washing
D. taking antibiotics

(489)

How long should a compounding pharmacy technician
scrub the hands and up to the elbow with warm water
and antimicrobial soap?

A. at least 30 to 90 seconds
B. at least 30 minutes
C. at least 5 minutes
D. at least 5 seconds

(490)

B. every 6 months

Rationale:

A compounder performing high-risk preparations should undergo validation testing every 6 months per USP 797. This ensures the competency of the technician compounding high-risk preparations.

(488)

C. hand-washing

Rationale:

Hand-washing is the most effective way to prevent contamination and the spread of infection within a hospital.

(489)

A. at least 30 to 90 seconds

Rationale:

A compounding pharmacy technician must scrub the hands and up to the elbow with warm water and antimicrobial soap for at least 30 to 90 seconds. Hand hygiene is important in preventing the spread of pathogens.

(490)

How often should all work surfaces and flooring of a cleanroom be sanitized?

A. every day
B. every week
C. twice per week
D. every month

(491)

At a minimum, how often should a pharmacy technician sanitize the walls and ceilings of a cleanroom?

A. daily
B. weekly
C. monthly
D. yearly

(492)

How often should a pharmacy technician sanitize the walls and ceilings of an anteroom?

A. daily
B. weekly
C. monthly
D. yearly

(493)

A. every day

Rationale:

All work surfaces and flooring of a cleanroom must be sanitized on a daily basis per USP 797 to eliminate contaminants.

(491)

C. monthly

Rationale:

The walls and ceilings of a cleanroom should be sanitized at least monthly per USP 797. Strict rules and procedures have to be followed to control contamination and reduce airborne particles within a cleanroom.

(492)

B. weekly

Rationale:

The walls and ceilings of an anteroom should be sanitized weekly per USP 797. The anteroom is the area outside the cleanroom where stock is stored and garbing takes place. Cleanliness of the anteroom is important to avoid contaminants from entering the cleanroom or contaminating individuals after garbing.

(493)

How long should the laminar airflow hood be turned on before use?

A. at least 5 minutes and it should be disinfected
B. at least 10 minutes and it should be disinfected
C. at least 20 minutes and it should be disinfected
D. at least 30 minutes and it should be disinfected

(494)

Which of the following is the proper garbing order?

A. head cover, face mask, beard cover (if needed), shoe covers, hand wash, gown, gloves
B. hand wash, head cover, face mask, beard cover (if needed), shoe covers, gown, gloves
C. gown, head cover, face mask, beard cover (if needed), shoe covers, hand wash, gloves
D. head cover, hand wash, face mask, beard cover (if needed), shoe covers, gown, gloves

(495)

D. at least 30 minutes and it should be disinfected

Rationale:

The laminar airflow hood should never be turned off. If turned off for any reason, it should be turned on for at least 30 minutes and disinfected before use.

(494)

A. head cover, face mask, beard cover (if needed), shoe covers, hand wash, gown, gloves

Rationale:

The proper garbing order is as follows: head cover, face mask, beard cover (if needed), shoe covers, hand wash, gown, and gloves. Following this garbing order is important to avoid contamination of hands after hand washing. For instance, if one hand washes first and then puts on the shoe cover, inevitably this person may touch his or her shoes and contaminate the hands.

(495)

How often should pharmacy balances be evaluated?

A. weekly
B. monthly
C. twice a year
D. once every year

(496)

What is the purpose of a breakdown room in a nuclear pharmacy?

A. quality control assurance of compounded radiopharmaceuticals
B. dispensing area of radiopharmaceuticals
C. restricted area where radiopharmaceutical returns or wastes are accepted
D. packaging area for delivery of radiopharmaceuticals

(497)

D. once every year

Rationale:

Pharmacy balances should be evaluated once every year. This is important to certify the proper functioning and efficiency of the balances.

(496)

C. restricted area where radiopharmaceutical returns or wastes are accepted

Rationale:

- The breakdown room of a nuclear pharmacy is a restricted area where radiopharmaceutical returns or wastes are accepted and broken down into different waste barrels.

- The quality control area is the location where quality assurance testing may be performed.

- The compounding area is the dispensing area.

- The packaging area is where radiopharmaceuticals are packaged for delivery.

(497)

Which of the following regulates the transport of hazardous materials?

A. the U.S. Department of Hazardous Materials
B. the U.S. Department of Transportation
C. the Environmental Protection Agency
D. the U.S. Department of Domestic Security

(498)

Which of the following United States Pharmacopeia (USP) chapters is related to compounding of hazardous drugs?

A. USP 61
B. USP 71
C. USP 797
D. USP 800

(499)

B. the U.S. Department of Transportation

Rationale:

The transport of hazardous materials (hazmat) is regulated by the U.S. Department of Transportation (USDOT). The Department of Transportation is concerned with loading, movement, and transport of wastes by all modes of transportation. It also regulates the specific types of waste containers, labels, markings, and vehicle placards. Transportation of hazmat is regulated by the Federal Hazardous Materials Transportation Law, which requires the training of all employees who will transport hazmat.

(498)

D. USP 800

Rationale:

USP 61 is related to microbiological examination of nonsterile products.

USP 71 is related to sterility tests.

USP 797 is related to compounding of sterile preparations.

Only USP 800 is related to compounding of hazardous drugs.

(499)

While on the job, a nurse calls with a question regarding the suitability of medical equipment for a given patient. What should the pharmacy technician do in this situation?

A. answer the nurse's question to the best of his or her knowledge
B. collect as much information as possible and search for the answer on the Internet
C. call the manufacturer of the medical equipment and share the nurse's concerns in hopes of finding the answer
D. direct the question to the pharmacist

(500)

D. direct the question to the pharmacist

Rationale:

All questions regarding medical equipment suitability should be directed to the pharmacist because they are better equipped to properly advise customers. Offering advice to customers on any medication-related inquiries and the suitability of medical devices is not within the pharmacy technician's scope of practice.

(500)

(Note: Numbers in the index refer to card numbers.)

Index

Index

Index

Index

Index

Index

Index

Index